THE
PREGNANCY
WORKBOOK

THE PREGNANCY
WORKBOOK

MANAGE ANXIETY AND WORRY WITH CBT AND MINDFULNESS TECHNIQUES

KATAYUNE KAENI, Psy.D., PMH-C

ROCKRIDGE
PRESS

Interior and Cover Designer: Elizabeth Zuhl
Art Producer: Janice Ackerman
Editor: Sean Newcott
Production Editor: Ruth Sakata Corley
Production Manager: Martin Worthington

Illustration: © Basia Stryjecka / Creative Market

Author Photo: Courtesy of Myke Aquino

ISBN: Print 978-1-64876-837-8 | eBook 978-1-64876-256-7
R1

I dedicate this book to my daughter Zella, whose birth threw me into the world of motherhood and into some of my deepest, most important work.

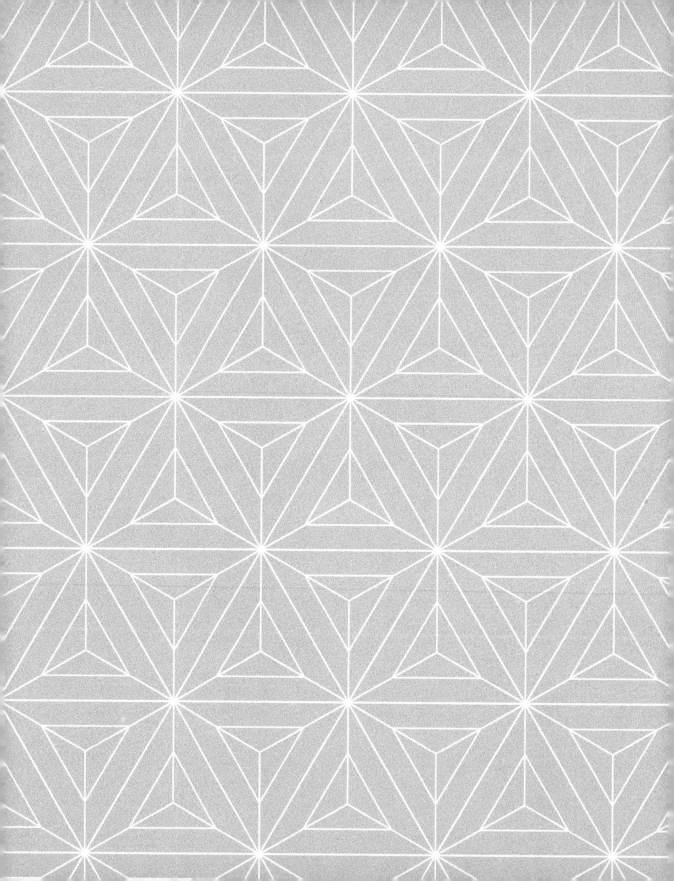

CONTENTS

Introduction viii

chapter one
Why Do I Feel This Way? 1

chapter two
Anxiety and Pregnancy 31

chapter three
Thought Modification 57

chapter four
Managing Distressing Thoughts 79

chapter five
Relaxation Techniques 99

chapter six
Mindfulness and Meditation 113

chapter seven
New Situation, New Strategies 127

chapter eight
Anxiety and Postpartum 141

chapter nine
Doing It Together 163

resources 179   references 183   index 187

INTRODUCTION

After the birth of my daughter, I was engulfed by a pain that I didn't know existed. Postpartum anxiety, postpartum depression, and postpartum obsessive-compulsive disorder took over my life for a year before I was able to figure out what was going on. I had never learned about these postpartum conditions, despite having been in the professional field of psychology for many years. Pregnancy, along with my devastating postpartum experience, ushered me into my life's work to educate and advocate for new parents' mental health.

For years now, I've specialized in perinatal mood and anxiety disorders and have supported many people through the transitions of conception, pregnancy, loss, birth, and postpartum. One of the most pervasive challenges people face is *not knowing*. Not knowing if they will get pregnant, stay pregnant, have a healthy baby, pregnancy, birth, or postpartum period. So many of the pregnant people I've supported just wanted to know that everything was going to be okay.

Many people are surprised to experience anxiety for the first time in pregnancy. After all, pregnancy is supposed to be a magical time, right? Pregnancy is filled with some magic for sure, but it can also present challenges for many people. If someone has a history of anxiety, they can be anxious in pregnancy, too. Furthermore, the process of trying to conceive, and the prospect of being pregnant, can be incredibly overwhelming for some. This is especially true if they have previously experienced a pregnancy loss.

Anxiety is common, and so are clinical levels of anxiety. But because anxiety is not often talked about, it can be very isolating, which, in turn, can produce more anxiety. Thankfully, people are working to change systems of care, adequately support new parents, and make sure people know that they are not alone. There's so much to know about the relationship between pregnancy and anxiety, and I'm hopeful that this workbook will help you feel more prepared and better supported.

How This Workbook Can Help

This workbook is focused on helping people who are experiencing anxiety for the first time during pregnancy as well as people who have a history of anxiety going into pregnancy, and will give you day-to-day coping skills to use before, during, and after pregnancy.

If no one told you that anxiety could be a part of pregnancy or having a baby, you're not alone. This workbook will shed light on the reality that many people experience and help you learn to notice your own physical, mental, and emotional cues about how you're feeling, then respond appropriately. That's what this book is for, to help you find ways to manage your feelings, self-soothe, find resources, and feel better.

This workbook will also address the ways in which anxiety can show up. I'll help you learn about anxiety, panic attacks, obsessive-compulsive disorder, post-traumatic stress disorder, and skills for coping with each. The symptoms of these conditions are important to be aware of, but the lived experience is much more nuanced and complex.

The tips, tricks, exercises, and skills in this workbook will come from many types of theoretical models of psychotherapy. I will be using an evidence-based approach, coming from a trauma- and resiliency-informed perspective. You will find cognitive behavioral therapy, dialectical behavior therapy, acceptance and commitment therapy, mindfulness strategies, and a great deal of information to help you on your journey.

It is important to know that as you read through the various anxiety conditions, your anxiety might increase—that is okay. But be sure to remind yourself that you don't need to take on any anxiety that isn't yours. You're already being proactive by using this workbook to learn and develop skills.

While you may see some of your experience reflected in this workbook, it can't cover every possible experience. If you don't see a specific symptom, thought, feeling, or behavior in this book, that doesn't mean your experience isn't real. It's real. It's valid. You're not imagining things, and you're certainly not alone. To that end, you will find many valuable resources at the back of this workbook to help you develop your coping skills as you continue on your pregnancy journey.

chapter one

Why Do I Feel This Way?

This chapter is ideal for someone who is pregnant and experiencing anxiety for the first time. Before unpacking this information, it's important to recognize that you didn't cause your anxiety and there's nothing wrong with you. There are reasons for your feelings. Anxiety can develop from one or several contributing factors related to your genetics, your body's response to hormonal changes, your current life situations, your past, or your concerns about the future.

As you complete this workbook, you're going to learn a lot about anxiety, but remember, that doesn't mean that everything will apply to you or that you'll experience everything that is discussed.

Pregnancy and Anxiety

Pregnancy can bring up many different feelings of worry and anxiety. You might be thinking, "Yes, it does for me, but that's just me. Other people seem to be fine." For perspective, consider this: Although different studies show varying prevalence rates, a research study in 2019 showed that having an anxiety disorder during pregnancy happens more often than previously thought, with rates being around one in five pregnancies. The study also showed a small tendency for anxiety to be slightly more common during pregnancy than during the postpartum period.

Because pregnancy is common, it comes with a specific myth that since other people do this all the time, it must be easy, predictable, and straightforward. Pregnancy is so highly valued in society that it carries myths that you will be fulfilled, feel beautiful, glow, and achieve a sense of purpose and meaning in the world. No pressure, right?

When it comes to your individual experience, you may feel pressure to be happy and grateful and hide any feelings of anxiety. Because of some of the myths surrounding pregnancy, you may feel like you can't or shouldn't have any negative feelings (or should not tell anyone about them if you do). And yet, here you are, feeling worried. Anxiety is real, so let's think about why that is the case.

You can't possibly predict what pregnancy is going to be like before it happens, which can cause anxiety. You can search the internet for answers to all of your questions, but in the end, your individual experiences are just that, individual. In addition, sometimes searching the internet for answers can give you *more* anxiety! Simple searches for information can reveal brand-new possibilities to worry about. You really can't know how pregnancy will affect you until you are going through it, but there are still some common worries.

Many of the anxieties I hear about from hopeful and pregnant parents are related to the fear of not knowing, which can make it feel like things are out of their control. Their anxieties sound a lot like this:

- *When will I get pregnant?*
- *How long will this take?*
- *What are these symptoms?*
- *Is this normal?*
- *How will my body change?*
- *What if I have a miscarriage?*
- *What if I do something that causes harm to the baby?*
- *How am I going to take care of a baby?*
- *How can I work when I feel so tired and sick?*
- *How will my partner handle this?*

When a person is pregnant, they aren't just thinking about themselves anymore. They have a new life that they are taking care of, sometimes happily, sometimes with great fear, sometimes both. Because of this, perinatal anxiety can focus on the baby or the health of the pregnancy. This added hypervigilance centered on the new life is very different from any other anxiety. It's anxiety for two.

The most important thing to know is that pre-conception and pregnancy anxiety is real. It's not just in your head, and you don't simply snap out of it. Anxiety is a real medical condition, and it deserves to be treated with the same respect as gestational diabetes or any other pregnancy complication. The myths of parenthood suggest that the parent is supposed to be nothing short of enthralled and blissful during pregnancy and with the new baby. The reality is that having a baby is a major life transition and comes with a mix of feelings, experiences, complexities, and emotional growth. Anxiety is more common than people think. The good news is that you don't have to be thrilled to be pregnant in order to be a good parent.

ANXIETY IN INFERTILITY AND PREGNANCY LOSS

Some common and understandable sources of anxiety are infertility and pregnancy loss. Infertility is defined as the body's inability to conceive a pregnancy after 12 months or more of continuous efforts with unprotected sex. When you're trying to conceive, every month brings a wide range of emotions, including nervousness, guarded hope and excitement, fear, sadness, guilt, and anger if there is no pregnancy. Sometimes anxiety about getting pregnant can stick around and become anxiety about staying pregnant.

Pregnancy loss happens for one in four pregnancies. Pregnancy loss is devastating and sometimes traumatic. For many people who have experienced pregnancy loss, fear of losing another pregnancy or something happening to the baby produces anxiety. The anxiety is real and to be expected because people don't want to experience another loss.

In most infertility and pregnancy loss situations, people feel a mix of reserved hope and worry about the baby, not wanting to connect fully to the idea of pregnancy or a baby in case something goes wrong. Sometimes people have a preoccupation with their own body. They may be hypervigilant about the signs and symptoms they are experiencing or want to hear the baby's heart rate frequently to make sure they are okay. If this is part of your anxiety experience, there are many resources available for support. Anxiety can feel very overwhelming and isolating. Know that you are not alone, and there is help. Please see the Resources section at the back of this workbook for ways you can find the support you need.

Wise Mind

The wise mind technique is a mindfulness skill used in dialectical behavior therapy (DBT) to help people find the middle ground between their emotional mind and their reasonable mind. This exercise can help you notice intense or excessive worry and name it as the emotional mind. It will also help you notice the part of your mind that is going over facts and details and name that as the reasonable mind. What would a balance be for you? How can you honor that balance to support reducing your worry?

EMOTIONAL MIND: Feelings are primary; thinking and behavior are controlled by emotions

REASONABLE MIND: Thinking is rational and logical

WISE MIND: A balance of emotion and logic; using intuition and logical thinking and experiencing emotion

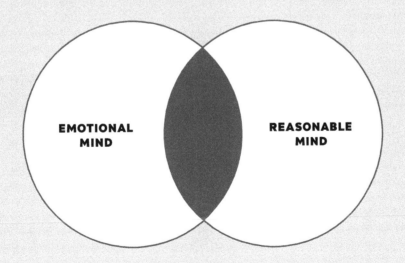

EMOTIONAL MIND

REASONABLE MIND

Making Sense of Your Thoughts and Emotions

I want to take a minute to point out a matter of great importance. It is essential for you to understand that having feelings of anxiety and having a clinical diagnosis of anxiety are two very different things.

Feelings of anxiety can show up in many ways, such as in emotions, thoughts, and bodily sensations. They might manifest as mild worry, tension in the body, restlessness, irritability, headache, gastrointestinal changes, nausea, or aches. The key is that the symptoms come and go or are relieved relatively easily when a situation improves or with adequate sleep, nutrition, and a connection with others.

A clinical diagnosis of anxiety in pregnancy is generally more impactful for a much longer time. Although the fundamental symptoms for antepartum anxiety are the same as those for generalized anxiety, the experiences and the reasons for the symptoms can be very different. In addition, anxiety can manifest in several different ways, such as panic attacks and obsessive-compulsive disorder (OCD). Anxiety can also manifest with other conditions, such as depression and post-traumatic stress disorder (PTSD).

So, how do you know when you're experiencing normal feelings of worry versus symptoms of anxiety at a clinical level? The answer is related to several factors.

LENGTH OF TIME. Think about how long you've been feeling anxious or worried. Has it been several days or several weeks? Several months? Do you feel anxious every day, or does the anxiety come and go occasionally? The length of time that your feelings or symptoms have been around is one of the indicators to keep track of as you go through pregnancy. Generally, experiencing anxiety or ongoing worry for several weeks or months is one sign that it is clinical.

With clinical anxiety, the worry feels out of control, like you can't really stop it from happening. You can also feel restless, tire easily, have difficulty concentrating, feel irritable, have tense muscles or body aches, or have difficulty falling or staying asleep.

ABILITY TO FUNCTION. Think about how you're getting through your days. Are you able to do most of the things you normally would? Is it getting difficult for you to do your day-to-day tasks because of the worry? Are you not doing the things you used to be able to do? Having a hard time functioning the way you used to is a potential indicator of a higher level of anxiety.

INTRUSIVE THOUGHTS. Sometimes high levels of anxiety can result in intrusive thoughts, which are sudden, scary, unwanted, and often related to the safety of the baby or yourself. Many people are taken aback by these thoughts, feel overwhelmed by them, and are confused as to why they would even have such thoughts. Intrusive thoughts can also feel obsessive, like you couldn't stop thinking about them even if you wanted to.

PANIC ATTACKS. Another way you can experience high anxiety is through a panic attack, which is a sudden, intense onset of fear that is often accompanied with a racing heart, trembling, difficulty breathing, lightheadedness, feeling like you're losing control, worry that you might die, or a feeling of being disconnected from things around you. A panic attack can last for 5 to 20 minutes and then subside.

Considering how much we've covered already, it may help to take a minute to consider your own pregnancy scenario, any symptoms you've noticed, and the presence of day-to-day anxiety in your life. To do so, let's take a closer look at your symptoms in the questionnaire below.

Your Anxiety Experience

Look over the following symptoms and questions and put a check next to the ones you're experiencing to better understand why you feel the way you do. Please note that this questionnaire is not a diagnosis or a complete professional assessment of your experience, and you may not personally experience one or even all of the symptoms described. Your answers can be used as a guidepost to help you access further help from a licensed health professional.

Anxiety

- Excessive anxiety and worry (more days than not for six months or more)
- Difficulty controlling the worry
- Feeling restless or fidgety
- Easily tired
- Difficulty concentrating
- Irritability
- Tension in your body
- Difficulty falling asleep or staying asleep

Are these symptoms affecting your ability to get through the day?

Panic Attack

- Heart racing
- Sweating
- Trembling
- Trouble catching your breath
- Feeling like you're choking
- Chest pain or pressure

- Nausea or diarrhea

- Dizziness or lightheadedness

- Feeling like the things around you are unreal

- Feeling like you're losing your mind

- Fear you might die

- Numbness or tingling in hands or feet

- Hot flashes or chills

Do these symptoms come on quickly and peak around 10 minutes?

Obsessive-Compulsive Disorder (OCD)

- Do you experience thoughts, impulses, or images that keep popping into your mind and seem intrusive and inappropriate? Do they cause you distress?

- Are those thoughts more than just everyday worries?

- Do you try to ignore or push out these thoughts, impulses, or images or try to make them stop by doing some other thought or action?

- Can you tell that the thoughts, impulses, or images are from your own mind (not put there by someone or something else)?

- Do you have repetitive physical or mental behaviors that you feel like you have to do when those thoughts or impulses come up in your mind? This behavior could be handwashing, counting, checking, repeating words, or something else that you feel like you have to do.

- Are you trying to prevent or reduce stress by doing this repetitive behavior?

- Does this response feel excessive or unreasonable to you?

CONTINUED ›

Your Anxiety Experience continued

○ Do the behaviors bother you or cause distress?

○ Do the behaviors take up a lot of your time or interrupt your routine or relationships?

Post-traumatic Stress Disorder (PTSD)

○ Did you witness or experience an event that threatened serious injury or death to you or someone else? (It could have been a perceived or actual threat.)

○ Did you feel intense helplessness or fear during this event?

○ Have you had recurrent distressing memories of the event?

○ Do you have any distressing dreams that keep coming back?

○ Does it ever feel like you're reliving the event?

○ Do you feel physically overwhelmed when you're reminded of the event or see something from it?

○ Do the same feelings you had during the event come up if you're reminded of it?

○ Do you try to avoid thoughts, feelings, people, places, or activities related to the event?

○ Is it hard to remember parts of what happened during the event?

○ Have you lost interest in things you used to enjoy?

○ Do you feel detached from people?

○ Is it hard to feel certain feelings?

○ Does it feel hard to see a possible future?

- Do you have any difficulties with sleep, anger, concentration, or feeling jumpy or on alert?

- Have you been feeling these things for more than a month?

- Have these feelings had an impact on your day-to-day life?

(List of symptoms taken from the fifth edition of the *Diagnostic and Statistical Manual of Mental Disorders: DSM-5*.)

Based on your responses to the questionnaire, you may fit into one or more categories. As a reminder, you may experience symptoms that don't fit into one diagnosis. Often, people experience symptoms that coincide with several diagnoses.

If you have several of these symptoms, please know that help is available and that you can feel better with the use of this workbook and the help of a qualified licensed mental health professional. Many people recover from these symptoms with the right help. You are not alone.

How Anxiety Can Be Expressed

Marissa found out she was pregnant but didn't feel ready to be a mom. She said that she might want to have a baby someday, but she wasn't ready right now. She had more that she wanted to do with her life and career before a baby arrived. She struggled because she did not like pregnancy, but she came to accept being pregnant and having a baby. Throughout the nine months, she worked on trying to wrap her mind around becoming a mother. She had a partner and planned on being with him for life, but they were struggling with the pregnancy news as a couple as well. She stated that she never "felt maternal" and wasn't sure if she would be a good mom, even though other people had always told her that they thought she would be. Her life was suddenly taking a new route that made her question herself all the time. "Am I going to be able to do this?" "What's going to happen to my body?" "Will my partner and I be able to stay together?" "How am I going to cope with the morning sickness and fatigue?"

One of the difficult things about anxiety is that it can be a very internal experience. People around you might not even be able to tell you are experiencing it. If you are like many people, you've likely been conditioned to keep your feelings inside and to show everyone that you have it all together. Yes, there's a time and place for doing that, but doing so all of the time can be very damaging to you.

Anxiety during pregnancy can feel like something that you have to hide, especially since the dominant narrative is that you are supposed to be happy that you are expecting. Believing and maintaining the myth of happiness is one of the reasons it can be hard to recognize when anxiety is present. If you feel like you have to deny the presence of anxiety, it can bring on a sense of shame or even guilt when you feel anxious.

In some cases, though, the anxiety can be so intense that it becomes more apparent to others than to yourself. That is why it is important to learn to recognize the signs and symptoms of anxiety. To help you do so, we will discuss some of the ways that anxiety can feel and look.

———

Anxiety puts your mind and body in a state of fear that can take several forms. Fight, flight, or freeze are the most common responses. These adaptive responses enable you to react when there is an emergency or a potentially threatening situation.

Imagine you're walking through a jungle and you step into a clearing and see a huge tiger in front of you. You are instinctually going to do what you need to do to survive, which would be to get ready to fight off a tiger attack, run away as fast as possible, or freeze to play dead or not be noticed. These responses are extremely useful when there's an emergency.

However, if your brain is responding to what-ifs or worst-case scenarios in the future and there isn't an actual tiger in front of you in that moment, then you're on alert for a possible emergency rather than an immediate emergency. It's true that there are things to worry about in pregnancy. It's not that you should never be anxious or worried. The key is to learn how to recognize anxiety and figure out how to manage it so that it doesn't feel like it's taking over.

In Marissa's story, several factors contributed to her anxiety.

1. Her pregnancy was not planned, expected, or initially wanted. This is a risk factor for perinatal mental health conditions in general, due to the huge upheaval unexpected pregnancy can bring. The prospect of putting your work on hold or making adjustments to your path can be a major stressor.

2. Marissa's pregnancy was physically and emotionally uncomfortable. Enduring a nine-month journey that she didn't really want to be on was a struggle. This contributed to her internal conflict of not wanting to be pregnant but trying to accept it, which made her further worry that she would not be ready to be a mother to this baby. The anxiety also heightened her concerns about not feeling maternal in the first place.

3. The strain on the relationship with her partner made her feel vulnerable that the relationship could end and she would have to figure out parenthood alone.

All of these factors are a part of the complex transition to parenthood, and it's enough to cause anyone to feel stress and anxiety. These feelings are by no means abnormal.

Let's look at ways that anxiety in pregnancy might be verbalized:

- *I'm supposed to be happy, so why do I feel anxious?*
- *I don't know what's going to happen. I can't stop worrying.*

- *Everybody else seems to be fine. Why aren't I?*
- *I tell people I'm excited because that's what you're supposed to say.*
- *I feel like I can't stop worrying about things.*
- *I'm tired, but I just can't sleep.*
- *My mind just keeps going and going.*

Some people may think or verbally express anxieties, while others may experience anxiety in pregnancy as a feeling. Some of these feelings may consist of the following:

WORRY. You may feel ongoing concern for many things.

IRRITABILITY. You may have feelings of irritation. They can be just under the surface, or you might be noticeably irritated with people and your surroundings. You might feel like any extra thing will overwhelm you.

RESTLESSNESS. You might feel fidgety, find it hard to sit and rest, need to get up and do things, or feel scattered.

PANIC. A panic attack sounds like what it feels like, panic. You can experience a sudden or unexpected state of high intensity that can include a rapid heart rate, sweating, dizziness or lightheadedness, nausea, tingling in your arms and legs, or tightness in your chest. You might also feel like you're choking or can't catch your breath, like you are having a heart attack, or like you're losing control or could die. You could become hyperfocused on how you're feeling and very worried that something bad is going to happen. Typically, these feelings last for 10 to 20 minutes and then begin to lessen.

DEEP SELF-DOUBT. You may have intense worry that you don't know what you're doing, that you aren't going to be able to be a parent, or that you made a decision and aren't sure if it's the right path. In pregnancy, self-doubt can show up as feeling like you can't handle things or even that you might fail.

CATASTROPHIC THINKING/WORST-CASE SCENARIO. Sometimes anxiety shows up by way of thinking of the worst outcome imaginable, or at least what would be the worst case for you. These thoughts, like many anxious thoughts, are irrational and lead people to think that the outcome will be worse than what is likely.

INTRUSIVE THOUGHTS/SCARY THOUGHTS. These types of anxiety-based thoughts feel like they come out of nowhere. They are very intense and feel terrifying or disturbing. They can even come with a visual of something terrible happening to you, your baby, or someone you love. Many types of intrusive thoughts are related to harm coming to you or your baby.

OBSESSIONAL THOUGHTS. These are thoughts, mental images, or feelings that are unwanted, cause distress, and feel overwhelming. The thoughts can be related to intense concerns about germs or cleanliness, such as intense worry about getting sick, or about harm coming to you or someone else. They might also manifest as being unsure or doubting that something happened or as intense, upsetting thoughts that you feel you can't stop. In pregnancy, these thoughts can feel like an ongoing and unwanted worry that something bad happened to the baby.

COMPULSIVE BEHAVIORS. Generally, compulsive behaviors develop as a result of obsessions and as a way to manage the intensity of anxiety. Compulsions are behaviors that you feel you must do in order to relieve yourself of the worry. For instance, you may worry about whether the baby's heart is beating, so you check it, and although you verify that it is beating, you still don't feel reassured, so you continue to check multiple times just to make sure.

OVERWHELM, NUMBNESS, OR INTENSE RESPONSES. Traumatizing events can leave you feeling out of sorts and not like yourself. You might think about the event often, try to not think about it at all, totally avoid it as much as possible, have bad dreams and recurring memories about it, feel disconnected from people around you, or even have difficulty remembering parts of the situation.

Self-Compassion

People often talk to themselves in negative and self-judgmental ways when they are going through times of stress, depression, and anxiety. Even though it's common, negative inner dialogue can do a lot of damage. If you're already feeling down or worried, making yourself feel bad about how you feel is like adding insult to injury, but because it's so common, you may not even know you are doing it to yourself.

In this exercise, you can reflect on how you talk to yourself. This thinking exercise is aimed to help you notice and be aware of your inner thought process, which gives you the opportunity to choose self-compassion rather than self-judgment.

1. When you feel overwhelmed and anxious, how do you talk to yourself?

2. Do you tell yourself that you should be happy?

3. Are you judgmental because you feel that you're not doing a good enough job?

4. If someone you love came to you and told you that they were going through the exact same thing you are going through, would you tell them that they should be happy? Would you tell them that they are not doing a good job?

5. If not, why wouldn't you say that to them?

6. Does how you talk to yourself seem mean or rude?

Remember to be kind to yourself. If you wouldn't say it to someone else, you don't need to say it to yourself. Practice what you could say to yourself by thinking of what supportive things you'd say to a friend. Then when you catch yourself being mean to yourself, say the supportive thing instead.

FEELING ANXIOUS

Somewhere along the way, we started to think about health and well-being in terms of mind or body. Your brain and body are actually very connected as part of a complex integrated system. Therefore, mental health issues are not just in your head. When you want to understand anxiety, you have to look at your entire system. It is not enough to just consider your emotions. You also must consider your thoughts, behaviors, and any physical manifestations. Since everyone's body responds differently to pregnancy, it can be useful to track your symptoms to see if they are related to anxiety or not. Here are some physical signs of anxiety to be mindful of:

GASTROINTESTINAL: Feeling nauseated or having diarrhea, heartburn, or a stomachache

RESTLESSNESS: Having difficulty sitting still or feeling fidgety, jittery, or on edge

HEART RACING: Feeling of your heart pounding inside your chest or beating quickly

SWEATING: Sweating relatively quickly on any part of your body, possibly for a short time

SHORTNESS OF BREATH OR SHALLOW BREATHING: Feeling like it's hard to catch your breath or that you can't get a full breath

MUSCLE TENSION: Feeling tension in your body, often in the shoulders, neck, back, or chest

DIFFICULTY WITH SLEEP: Having problems falling asleep or staying asleep, leading to tiredness during the day

Sharing Your Feelings

Finding a way to talk to your partner, family, or friends about the changes in your mood can be challenging. Sharing our thoughts and feelings about anxiety or other mood changes in pregnancy can make us feel vulnerable. Therefore, it's important to find people you can trust with your feelings and who will listen to you without judgment. Being anxious in pregnancy is hard, but it's harder to feel anxious and alone.

Relationship dynamics can change with fertility, pregnancy, and postpartum complications. This is a common but major stressor for many people. Know that this is perfectly normal, but it's also important during this time to seek out professional psychotherapy services to help figure things out, either individually or with your partner.

If you have a partner and would like for them to learn more about how they can support you, send them on over to chapter 9. There, they can find tips on how to be supportive, how to communicate, and how to notice their own stress and need for self-care.

Now, let's go over some tips and strategies for communicating your symptoms, feelings, and needs.

Talking with Your Partner

Talking with your partner about anxious feelings and mood changes can range from very easy to very difficult depending on your relationship and style of communication. This workbook can help you understand how you're feeling so that it's easier to explain to others. But sometimes you don't know how you're feeling, and that's okay, too. Feelings are funny that way. They don't always make themselves clear from the get-go. Ideally, you can talk about that with your partner as well.

---

tip

When your partner asks you how you're doing, if you're not fine, try not to say that you're fine. Instead, you can say, "I don't know yet, but when it's clear to me, I'll let you know."

If there is difficulty or tension in your relationship, it can be difficult to open up. Sometimes you have to gauge for yourself whether it's a good time to talk about your vulnerable feelings. Some partners don't understand anxiety, or pregnancy for that matter. I often hear from people in difficult relationships that they don't want their partner to know what's going on because it's more of a hassle. They want to protect themselves from having their feelings minimized or invalidated altogether. These are very real challenges. Sometimes communicating about feelings is easier with a friend or family member.

If it's easy to communicate with your partner, sharing how you're feeling can be a regular part of checking in with each other. Let's look at some realities about talking with your partner.

IT CAN BE HARD TO KNOW WHAT YOU FEEL OR HOW TO EXPRESS YOUR FEELINGS. You can say that out loud, too. Telling your partner that you haven't figured out how you are feeling is part of communication. Your feelings don't have to be in a neat little package. Sometimes you may figure out your feelings *while* you are talking about them. Just do the best that you can with the information you have so far.

YOU DON'T HAVE TO KNOW WHAT YOU NEED YET. Yes, you read that right. It's okay to not know. Often, partners are in "fix it" mode. They want to know clearly what they can do to help and may not understand why you don't know yet. Communicating that you will tell them when you understand your needs better can reduce some of the anxiety about having to come up with answers and explanations.

TELL YOUR PARTNER HOW THEY CAN HELP. Your partner can't do everything for you, but if you have a clear sense of what you need from them, that would be a great help. I often hear from clients that they wish their partner would just know what to do and then do it. Unless your partner is psychic, you probably will have to spell it out for them. And even after that, they might not be able to do what you need when you need it. I suggest having an idea of what you need and asking them what they can do based on that.

KNOW THAT YOUR PARTNER MAY BE HAVING FEELINGS, TOO. You are the pregnant person. You are carrying the child and dealing with all of the physical and emotional effects of pregnancy. However, your partner is also going through a change. They are becoming a parent, too, and they may need their own support. They may not be feeling the same intensity of anxiety that you are, but then again, they might be. Partners can also experience clinical anxiety or depression during this period of time. We will talk more about that in chapter 9.

Keeping Connection Together

▼

The journey into parenthood can be something that brings a couple together, but it can also contribute to feeling disconnected. Life gets busy, and you may not have a lot of time together due to work or other scheduling restrictions. In addition, each partner may have a different view of, or feelings about, pregnancy and welcoming a child. There are many ways that disconnection can affect a couple.

One way to keep the connection is to schedule time to check in every week. As a couple, you might have some specific things to talk about, but here are some general questions to ask each other.

- *How are you feeling this week?*
- *What are some positives or wins personally or in our relationship?*
- *What are some difficulties you've encountered personally or in our relationship?*
- *What are some individual needs that you have for this week?*
- *How can I support you?*

Talking with Other Family Members

Some of your family members may be able to relate to the feelings that you're having. They might not have called it anxiety during their pregnancies because there wasn't a wide understanding of perinatal mood and anxiety disorders a generation ago. There may be others in your family who simply do not understand why you feel anxious. They may even minimize your feelings or tell you that you're overreacting. If someone has not gone through what you're going through, they may not be able to respond with sympathy.

Some of the tips for talking with partners apply to talking with family members. However, there may be other complicating factors when communicating with family, depending on your relationship history, culture and ethnicity, traditions, religion or spirituality, family history, or family expectations. These are all highly nuanced situations, so I will offer some basic ideas for communication. I would urge you to seek out culturally relevant guidance from a trusted family member, friend, or elder to help with more specific concerns.

One specific difference with family that I see is that they tend to have a lot of advice to give. Sometimes that advice is supportive and feels great. Other times that advice can feel overbearing, intrusive, or very different from how you are choosing to be pregnant.

Again, depending on your family culture, you may be able to express that the advice is overwhelming or that you don't want support in that way. For some families, listening to your elders or even seeking out their guidance is expected, especially when it comes to pregnancy and childrearing. These family and cultural dynamics can be difficult if you as the pregnant person are the first or even the second generation in a different country of origin than that of your parents. Differing ideas of how to care for a pregnancy and how to raise a child can come with conflict.

If your family system is generally supportive or doesn't contribute to your anxiety, it can be a source of stability and reliability. Most family systems have a mix of ease and difficulty, love and conflict, closeness and distance. Having the support of a partner or a friend can help ease any stress that is associated with family.

Talking with Friends

Social support is one of the key factors in coping with a perinatal mood or anxiety disorder. Having friends who really understand what you're feeling can be a major relief. As you may have already gathered, not everyone will understand or be supportive.

If you can, find at least one person you can be honest with. Being able to talk about your feelings can relieve the stress and pressure that you might be feeling. Talking with a friend can be a little less complicated than talking with a partner or family member because the friend might be able to be more objective.

If you can't find that one person in your group of friends, you can seek out a support group of other pregnant people. Pregnancy and postpartum support groups, both online and locally, can offer a safe space to talk about feelings. Some of those groups are listed in the Resources section of this workbook.

Communication

▼

If you feel overwhelmed by the idea of talking with your partner, family, or friends about your pregnancy concerns, write out how you feel first. Writing can help you gather your thoughts and focus on what's most important to you. Anxiety, specifically, makes you worry, and that can sidetrack your original goal of reaching out for connection and support during pregnancy.

Begin by centering your thoughts on your desired conversation about staying connected. Then, go through the questions below to support you in your communication process.

1. What am I experiencing? Include feelings, thoughts, concerns, and physical sensations.

2. What do I want my partner, family member, or friend to understand about what I'm experiencing?

3. What kind of support do I need?

4. How would I like to receive that support from my partner, family member, or friend?

Seeking Professional Support

You don't need to be suffering in order to justify reaching out for help. Seeking professional services from a psychotherapist isn't a sign of weakness. It doesn't mean you've failed, it doesn't mean you couldn't figure it out on your own, and it certainly doesn't mean that it's "all in your head." These are all reasons I've heard people give for why they didn't get help sooner. They ended up suffering far longer than they needed to because of the stigma around mental health issues.

The great news is that anxiety in pregnancy is treatable. You can actually feel better with the right kind of help. The field of perinatal mental health is continuing to emerge as a necessary specialty in mental healthcare. There are now thousands of therapists who have specialized training in perinatal mood and anxiety disorders, the mental health transition to parenthood, and how to support parents adjusting to life with a baby. Within this specialty, there are other specializations that are particularly supportive for people wanting to be pregnant, for people who are pregnant, and for those who have experienced a loss or have a new baby.

If you've never been to therapy or sought out a therapist, it can be a daunting and intimidating process. I'm going to help demystify the process. There are many types of psychotherapists, and they may have one of many types of professional degrees. Some psychiatrists also do psychotherapy; however, many of them focus on assessment and treatment with psychotropic medications.

There are master's clinicians:

- LCSW (licensed clinical social worker)
- MFT/LMFT (licensed marriage and family therapist)
- LPCC (licensed professional clinical counselor)
- Other master's license types, depending on the state you're in

There are also doctoral clinicians:

- Psy.D. (doctor of psychology)
- Ph.D. (doctor of philosophy)

LOOK FOR PERINATAL MENTAL HEALTH SPECIALISTS. For perinatal clients, I highly suggest finding a therapist who specializes in perinatal mental health. Therapists who are perinatal mental health certified (PMH-C) have the foundational training necessary to adequately support, diagnose, and treat conditions. They can also tell you if referral to additional specialists would be beneficial. It's important to ask a potential therapist if they have specific training in perinatal mental health or maternal mental health. Although therapists can be supportive without this training, a specialist will be familiar with many different complexities and diagnoses, which will help them better identify what is going on with you. The role of a perinatal mental health certification is to make sure that new parents are getting a professional who has solid knowledge of perinatal mood and anxiety disorders.

Here are some tips for finding a therapist:

GET A PERSONAL RECOMMENDATION. Find out if someone you know can give you a personal recommendation.

SEARCH THE INTERNET. You can do an internet search for the kind of therapist you're looking for, such as "pregnancy anxiety therapist." You can also consult an online therapy directory, which will allow you to search for a therapist near you or in your state. Many of the directories have filters, such as gender, insurances accepted, types of issues the therapist helps with, types of therapy they have training in, and specific populations they work with, to help narrow down your search.

FIND SEVERAL OPTIONS. I suggest that you find several therapists who look like they might be a good fit for you. The list doesn't have to be lengthy, but having options is always a good thing.

CONTACT THEM. Let them know briefly what is going on, what you'd like help with, and ask any questions you have for them about how they work and whether they can help with your needs.

KEEP GOING UNTIL YOU FIND THE RIGHT FIT. Finding a therapist that is a good fit for you is very important. Continue your search until you find someone you feel you can trust and who will listen and understand your situation.

SCHEDULE AN APPOINTMENT. Once you set the initial appointment with the therapist, generally there will be some documents to review about starting therapy, office policies, and one or more questionnaires to fill out.

ATTEND YOUR FIRST SESSION. In your first session, the therapist will try to understand your situation as much as possible, so they may have questions for you or just ask you to share more about why you want to begin therapy.

Speaking of therapy, there are over 400 types of psychotherapy! Different types of therapy work for different people. The following list includes some of the types that are used to support perinatal mental health for individuals or couples.

COGNITIVE BEHAVIORAL THERAPY (CBT). CBT looks to incorporate how you think, feel, and behave to understand how your distress is affecting you. This form of therapy makes clear how your stressors affect your thoughts, feelings, and behavior, then takes those factors into consideration when determining which skills could be helpful in your process of healing. CBT includes learning relaxation skills and how to label cognitive distortions, modify anxious thoughts, challenge negative thinking, and generate alternatives to negative thoughts. The therapist will often give practice work for the client to do between sessions.

INTERPERSONAL PSYCHOTHERAPY (IPT). IPT is a time-limited therapy that is helpful for interpersonal issues. Its goals are to reduce symptoms of mood disorders, improve interpersonal relationships, and increase social functioning. This therapy focuses on resolving interpersonal deficits, building social connection, and managing grief, life transitions such as divorce or parenthood, and interpersonal disputes.

ACCEPTANCE AND COMMITMENT THERAPY (ACT). ACT is a form of therapy that helps people learn to accept difficult thoughts and feelings that may actually be appropriate responses to stressful and challenging situations, all while working toward healthy change. This therapy helps you embrace your thoughts and feelings instead of suppressing them or feeling guilty about them.

EYE MOVEMENT DESENSITIZATION AND REPROCESSING (EMDR). EMDR is a therapy that reduces the emotional distress related to traumatic memories and experiences. It helps you process thoughts, memories, and feelings that feel stuck or hard to resolve so that you can feel less overwhelmed by the difficult experiences you've had. This therapy uses back-and-forth eye movement and alternate side to side tapping of the arms or legs, or alternating left/right sounds in a fast pace, while the person recalls aspects of the difficult or traumatic situation. This technique, along with the therapist guiding you, lets you process the trauma and helps it to not feel as intense.

Psychotropic medication can also be greatly beneficial when symptoms become disruptive to daily life. Chapter 2 will go more in depth about using medication before, during, and after pregnancy.

Search for a Therapist

Searching for a therapist can feel overwhelming, especially if you haven't looked for one before. There are many types of therapy and many reasons that people seek the support of psychotherapy. You don't have to know exactly what you need before you reach out to a therapist. Sometimes therapy is where you figure out what you need. Therapists are trained to help people gain clarity and develop coping skills.

Many therapists will talk with you for 10 to 15 minutes to see if they can help your specific situation before setting up an initial appointment. You can tell them why you're interested in therapy and ask them questions about how they can help. You can use online therapist directories to help refine your search for a therapist. It's important to find one who is a good fit for you. You might need to try out a couple of them to get a feel for the working relationship.

In the following exercise, you can start to think through what you might want or need out of psychotherapy. Use the parameters that are listed to start thinking about what might be important to you. Then, list for yourself a few more details about what you'd like to get from psychotherapy. This list can help you have a conversation with the therapists you reach out to.

Issues you want to address

Type of license

CONTINUED ▸

Search for a Therapist continued

Racial or ethnic identity

_____

Trauma informed

_____

Social justice informed

_____

Insurances accepted

_____

Private pay (and range you can afford)

_____

Type of therapy you prefer (if known)

_____

Virtual or in person

_____

Sexuality or gender of therapist

_____

Spiritual identity/knowledge

_____

PEOPLE DON'T ALWAYS SAY THE RIGHT THING

People have a lot of opinions and advice related to conception and pregnancy. You're going to hear things that are wrong, offensive, or inappropriate. Usually, people are trying to connect with you or relate something they heard. Sometimes these comments are okay, but sometimes they can be hurtful. For instance, when I was pregnant, I walked into a work meeting and someone yelled across the room, in front of all of my coworkers, "You look like a bowling pin!" I've also heard, "Are you having twins? You're huge!" People give out medical advice, their opinions on baby names, horror stories they've heard, bad experiences they've had, and much more. The best thing you can do for yourself, aside from setting healthy boundaries, is to try to not take these comments personally, which would add to your already anxious state.

Setting a boundary can be challenging, and it may need to be altered depending on who you're talking with. Some elements of boundary dynamics include:

1. You don't like what's being done or said.
2. The crossing of the boundary affects your relationship with that person.
3. They might be unaware that it's affecting you.
4. You might be concerned that setting a boundary will make the other person upset.
5. Not saying something will continue to affect you.

There are ways to address boundary crossing in the moment:

- A diplomatic verbal response, for example, could be, "I know you're being funny, but I'd rather not hear those types of jokes about my body."
- A response to unsolicited advice could be something like, "Thanks for your thoughts/concerns/ideas, but that won't/doesn't work for me."
- Sometimes you'll need to be more direct by just saying, "Please stop" or "No thanks."

chapter two

Anxiety and Pregnancy

When you have anxiety or a history of anxiety, becoming pregnant might make your symptoms return or heighten them. A history of a mental health condition is a risk factor for the condition returning or worsening in pregnancy or the postpartum period, but the good news is that with a workbook like this, you can work on a plan of care that can help you manage anxiety.

Anxiety, by its nature, makes you worry about the future and makes you want to manage as many of your concerns as possible. Pregnancy also naturally comes with a lot of unknowns. Wanting to manage something that you've never experienced can feel like a huge challenge. Sometimes you can't make anxiety come to a complete stop, but you can certainly find ways to manage the intensity of it and feel better.

On the Way to Pregnancy

The overall path to pregnancy can be a long and winding road. Sometimes it can take a while to become pregnant. Sometimes pregnancy can come about quickly. The longer the path, the more decisions you may have to make about how to move forward. In any case, the decision-making process will begin, but it's more than that—your path to parenthood is beginning, too.

Ambivalence Is Okay

Becoming a parent is an emotional, physical, mental, and sometimes spiritual process. Feeling unsure is part of any growing process. It's pretty normal to go back and forth in your mind about how you feel in regard to the pregnancy and parenthood, whether it's a subtle questioning of your decision or outright anxiety about the path you're on. I am not sure where the pressure to be 100 percent all in and happy comes from, but I can tell you that it often contributes to anxiety and shame. If you don't continue to try to normalize that there is a full, complex, and very normal set of conflicted feelings about pregnancy and parenting, you will continue to secretly carry anxiety and shame.

The Ups and Downs with Each Month of Trying

People who are on the path to get pregnant often describe the roller coaster of emotions that can come with each month of anticipation, hopefulness, and nervousness about whether they will be pregnant or not. If pregnancy doesn't come that month, there can be a disappointment and sadness that feels a bit like grief. Then they begin gearing up to try again, hoping for the best and fearing the worst. Months of these ups and downs can lead to anxiety, frustration, sadness, anger, and sometimes distrust of one's own body.

Becoming Pregnant

Becoming pregnant can be a very joyous and exciting time. If you wanted to be pregnant and became pregnant, the goals and hopes you had for a family are that much closer. However, for some people, a confirmation of pregnancy is not actually exciting. That may seem surprising, but it's common. Pregnancy can come with many emotional reactions, some of which might surprise you. People who have been trying to become and stay pregnant for a while might feel a responsibility or gravity about pregnancy that they didn't anticipate having.

Sometimes people who wanted pregnancy were anxious when it happened sooner than they expected. If you have a history of anxiety, pregnancy can bring up new anxieties or intensify anxiety that was already there.

Worry about Body Changes

Jenny had struggled with negative body image since her teenage years. In her adult life before becoming pregnant, she was very focused on working out and monitoring her food intake, and she was hyper-aware of any new changes in her body. Once she became pregnant, the worry about how her body would change started to set in. In the early months, she "felt fat" and didn't like how she was feeling physically. She described feeling overwhelmed, like her body was doing things that she couldn't control, like gaining weight, feeling bigger, and feeling tired and nauseated. She didn't like pregnancy because of all of this. She went to the gym more often, had anxiety about being weighed at the doctor's office at each checkup, and generally felt bad about herself due to the body changes.

Terry, on the other hand, was happy to be pregnant but had mixed feelings about their body changes during pregnancy. They had lived in a larger body most of their life and had many encounters with medical staff about body and weight that felt invalidating. Furthermore, they were worried that they wouldn't look pregnant to others. Although they felt comfortable in their body, the pressure of other people's perceptions created stress.

Your body is pretty amazing. In pregnancy, you grow a person and a whole other organ (the placenta), your blood volume increases, your uterus expands, and your belly and skin grow and stretch to accommodate new life. It just happens. You don't have to do anything for the amazing transformation to take place. Your thought processes and emotions expand, and your sense of self adapts over time. People who have had difficult relationships with their bodies in the past or who have body image concerns during pregnancy can feel increased anxiety. There are countless ways that you can relate to your body depending on culture, societal pressures, family dynamics, history of physical trauma, body size, physical abilities, or any number of other factors. Many people feel concerned about the outward appearance of their body, pressured to not gain too much weight and to stay fit, concerned about how medical providers will treat someone living in a larger body, and self-conscious about how their pregnant body looks.

"I Don't Care What the Sex of the Baby Is, As Long As It's Healthy"

While many people really may feel neutral about whether their baby is assigned male or female at birth, some people really do care about the sex of their baby. In fact, when the sex of the baby is not what the parent wanted, it can be anxiety producing, depressing, or even devastating for them. This disappointment is complex. It may not be apparent to anyone else but the gestational parent or their partner, and it can happen regardless of whether they find out the assigned sex during pregnancy or when the baby is born. For some people finding out during pregnancy gives them time to process or grieve before the baby arrives. Let's look at a couple of examples.

MONICA. Monica was really hoping for a girl because she grew up in a family of girls. She felt that she didn't know how to raise a boy or how to relate to one. This feeling brought up a fear that she wouldn't be able to connect with her son, and that fear contributed to her feeling disconnected from her son during the pregnancy.

ROYA. Roya didn't want to have a girl because of her own history of unhealed trauma. She felt it would be easier to have a boy that she wouldn't have to worry about.

ZOE. Zoe was the first among their siblings to have a baby. Culturally, their elders' preference was for the first child to be a boy. Zoe felt immense pressure to not disappoint the family, even though Zoe didn't agree with the cultural norm.

Worry about Birth

The concept of growing a human inside your body, then bringing them out from your body by vaginal delivery or C-section can be a mind-bending concept. Yes, people have done it since the beginning of time, but this is your experience, and

Reflection and Developing Compassion

▼

In many ways, healing begins with awareness. You cannot attend to things you are not aware of in your mind or body. Body awareness can be a difficult process to start, as many people may feel disconnected from their bodies or hyperaware of them. Gauge for yourself how it feels to consider the following questions, and if it's overwhelming, then you have that information and can come back to this when you are ready.

As you consider the questions, do so with gentleness and the intention to understand yourself more deeply. This exercise may be helpful and even surprise you in terms of what your reflection brings up. You can answer the questions in your mind or use them as journaling prompts.

1. *What is the state of my relationship with my body?*

2. *How do I feel about my body becoming and being pregnant?*

3. *What fears do I have about my body in pregnancy?*

4. *In what ways has my body been resilient?*

5. *In what ways can I honor the work my body does to keep me going?*

6. *Are there things about my body that I can feel good about during this pregnancy?*

it's unique to you. For people who worry or have clinical anxiety related to birth, there's a range of concerns.

One concern is the anticipation of pain and how they are going to handle that pain. It's pretty hard to try to imagine something like a vaginal birth or a C-section if you've never experienced it. There's nothing to compare that to, so the worry can be all over the place. I hear a lot of clients express self-doubt about vaginal birth. They wonder if they can do it and how they will handle it. What I can tell you is that worry doesn't really help your confidence, yet people still birth their children. You'll know after the baby is out that you can do it.

Another worry is that you won't or can't have the birth that you prefer. Even with a plan or birthing wishes in place, there is an element of unknown in the birthing process, which can increase worry. People don't worry about the process going well or okay. They worry about it going badly. For a few people, this fear of birth and pregnancy is so intense that it becomes a phobia called tokophobia, the fear of pregnancy and childbirth.

In addition to needing to learn about the birth itself, there is a lot of pressure to develop a birth plan: how you want to get your baby out, what interventions you want (or don't want) from a medical care team, where you want to give birth, who you want in the room with you, and so on. Depending on how your anxiety is playing out, you can range from wanting to just get the baby out safely to wanting to control as many things as possible. Let me just say, it's reasonable to want to control things. This is your child, and you are already parenting by wanting to keep them safe. Still, you can't control everything, and it can be hard to handle this realization. The compromise is to plan for what you can control and be flexible with what you can't, which is more like a mix of a birth *plan* and birth *hopes*. For instance, you can communicate your expectations and preferences about procedures, medications, and postpartum care for you and for the baby while also staying flexible mentally. Staying flexible rather than having rigid expectations helps you cope with whatever changes come with the birthing and postpartum process.

The Internet Doesn't Always Know Best

Let's get real about internet research. It's not always your friend. Your anxiety might want answers. With information at your fingertips, it's very easy to type in your question and send it out into the ether and see what comes back.

Sometimes what may seem like an answer for you is someone else's experience, which may or may not be supportive to you. Time and time again, I hear from clients about how they dive in for answers and find more things to be worried about.

There's nothing inherently wrong about looking for answers online, but temper the searching by remembering that your personal experience is valid. Sometimes setting time limits or even limiting the number of clicks to adjoining articles can help manage the pull down the rabbit hole.

Finding a Team of Providers

There are many options for providers who can support you with self-care and help with mental and physical distress management. Let's look at the types of providers that can assist you with your pregnancy process. Please consult with your primary care provider to see if the options are appropriate for your situation.

OB-GYN: Physician who assists with pregnancy, childbirth, and medical conditions related to reproductive organs

MIDWIFE: A person who's trained to assist in pregnancy and childbirth and provides prenatal and postpartum care

NURSE MIDWIFE: Registered nurse who has additional training to assist in pregnancy and childbirth and provides prenatal and postpartum care

BIRTH OR POSTPARTUM DOULA: A person who provides physical and emotional support during childbirth and/or postpartum care after the baby comes home

PERINATAL OR MATERNAL MENTAL HEALTH PSYCHOTHERAPIST: A therapist who provides counseling and support related to fertility, pregnancy, loss, birth, and postpartum

REPRODUCTIVE PSYCHIATRIST: A specialist psychiatrist who understands pregnancy and postpartum and can prescribe psychiatric medications

PREGNANCY SUPPORT GROUP: A support group of people who are experiencing similar struggles

LACTATION CONSULTANT: A person trained to help with breastfeeding

Anxiety Is Overwhelming

Anxiety has a way of jumbling up your mind so that it's hard to settle down, which can make you feel like you are in an anxiety spiral: a perpetual cycle of what-ifs, worries, and uncertainty.

Let's break it down a little so that you can get a sense of what you're really worried about. But before that, it is important to remember your strengths. You've made it this far in life and have surely figured out some creative ways to cope.

1. What are your strengths?

2. What are the coping skills you've already learned?

3. Are they still working for you?

4. What are your concerns or fears in general?

5. List your concerns about trying to become pregnant.

6. List your concerns about being pregnant.

7. Do you have concerns about birth?

8. Do you have concerns about postpartum?

Now that you have your concerns in a little more focus, how does it feel to see them on paper? Does it seem like the skills you have can help with these? If not, look into the following chapters for more skills and tools. Do you feel like more support from a professional would be helpful? See chapter 1 for ideas on how to find a therapist that specializes in perinatal mental health.

ACUPUNCTURE: A component of traditional Chinese medicine in which fine therapeutic needles are superficially inserted into the skin at specific points to foster healing

CHIROPRACTOR: A person with training in how to support the nervous system and align the musculoskeletal systems

LICENSED NATUROPATHIC DOCTOR: A physician who treats chronic and acute illness holistically by supporting a person's self-healing processes

HOSPITAL: Conventional place for labor and delivery

BIRTHING CENTER: A facility for birthing staffed by midwifes, OB-GYNs, nurses, and doulas

PELVIC FLOOR PHYSICAL THERAPIST: A provider who treats the muscles, nerves, and connective tissues of the pelvic floor and region

PRENATAL MASSAGE: A type of massage specifically for pregnancy that supports muscle relaxation

Depending on any previous medical conditions, your pregnancy care provider may suggest other needed or supportive treatment providers and options.

ANXIETY AND DEPRESSION

It is common for people to experience anxiety and depression at the same time. One can affect or bring on the other. Both can manifest as irritability, difficulty concentrating, and changes in sleeping and eating habits. For some people, the two conditions together can cause an agitated depression that includes feelings of intense anger or rage. Clinical depression consists of a sad mood, low motivation, lack of interest in things you used to enjoy, feeling bad about yourself, and, when severe, thoughts of death or suicide. Experiencing several of these symptoms consecutively for more than two weeks may be a sign of depression. Please reach out to your care team to discuss options for support.

Medication and Pregnancy

Psychotropic medication during pregnancy can be a hot-button issue. There are a lot of opinions and misconceptions, as well as some risk. But there are highly trained and specialized reproductive psychiatrists and nurse practitioners who are equipped to evaluate a perinatal person's prescription needs. Thankfully, many other physicians and prescribing professionals are receiving advanced training in reproductive psychiatry to be better equipped to support pregnant people.

As a psychologist, I cannot prescribe or recommend specific medications, but I can give you a general introduction to the idea of medication during pregnancy and the types of medications that are generally known to treat anxiety during the perinatal period. I will provide you with resources that can help you locate a provider or more clinical information.

In my practice, I've had a wide range of experience with clients, from those who want to try everything possible to avoid psychiatric medication to those who say that there is no way they will stop taking their medication because life is worse without it. There is always a choice to take or not to take medication, but for some people, it's a necessity. For some people, it's a lifesaver.

There's an interesting phenomenon that happens with psychiatric medications that doesn't happen as often with medications for other medical conditions. The way that mental health is stigmatized more so than physical health plays into the way that medication is perceived.

For instance, if someone has diabetes and needs to take insulin, no one questions it at all. However, when someone has anxiety or depression, sometimes they are told that they should "get over it" or "snap out of it." Clinical anxiety is a medical condition, too. People can't just choose to be done with it. If it were that easy, they would have done it already. So, just like mild forms of diabetes, mild anxiety can be managed with diet, exercise, and self-care. When it's moderate to severe, though, medication is sometimes required, just as it is for moderate to severe physical issues.

Taking medication while pregnant, however, comes with more concern and scrutiny, and rightly so. Thankfully, much research is being conducted to determine the effects of medication on pregnancy and babies. Ongoing research of medications in pregnancy is helping provide guidance as to what is safe and what is not.

Risk of Medication vs. Risk of Untreated Medical Condition

There is reasonable concern with taking any medication during pregnancy. Anecdotally, there seems to be an even more heightened concern about taking medication for anxiety or depression in pregnancy. There is considerable stigma around mental health and medication in general, and when you add in pregnancy, it becomes a hot-button issue. Common worries are related to the development of the baby in utero. It's an understandable concern and one that should be closely considered with the support of your OB-GYN, midwife, psychiatrist, or nurse practitioner. Most practitioners who prescribe medication use a risk-versus-benefit decision-making process.

What a lot of people don't know is that untreated anxiety or any other moderate to severe mental health condition also carries risk to the baby in utero. This is a particularly hard fact for pregnant people who experience anxiety because when they learn that high levels of anxiety for longer stretches of time affect the baby, they can feel guilty. They can feel stuck, as if no decision they make is good. They just have to make the best decision they can with the information they have and the help of their medical providers.

What a lot of people and providers don't know is that if you are on medication already, it may be safe to continue it. You or your provider should consult a reproductive psychiatrist. Unfortunately, I've seen far too many people quit medication cold turkey and have rebound symptoms that make their anxiety worse. The pregnant person and their baby are made more vulnerable to the symptoms of anxiety when medication is stopped abruptly.

There are several types of medications that are commonly used for anxiety, obsessive-compulsive disorder (OCD), panic, and depression. Benzodiazepines are short-acting medications, used as needed when anxiety peaks. Other daily use medications often fall into the antidepressant category and are commonly used for anxiety as well. Depending on your history or family history, your physician may suggest these or other types of medications after considering the risk versus the benefit to you.

tip

Thyroid function can change in pregnancy. Hypothyroidism can come with mood changes such as depression. It can also cause fatigue and make you feel slow. Hyperthyroidism symptoms can include anxiety, mental restlessness, and a higher heart rate. You can ask your medical care provider about thyroid testing.

Your Medical Conditions and Medications

▼

Make a list of your medical conditions, medications and dosages, and any supplements you are currently taking. This can be a useful list to take to a provider when seeking a medication evaluation. Please include supplements when talking with your medical provider so that they can determine if a new medication has any contraindications with the supplements or other medications you are currently taking.

MEDICAL CONDITION	MEDICATION	DOSAGE

SUPPLEMENTS:

SLEEP IS MAGIC

All conditions can worsen without adequate sleep. Sleep should be a major part of any self-care plan before, during, and after a pregnancy. The brain and body need sleep to feel restored and to function well. Anxiety can make falling asleep and staying asleep challenging. This, on top of all the physical changes your body experiences as your baby grows, can cause insomnia in pregnancy, which can worsen an underlying anxiety or create its own anxiety. Please consult with your care team about how to ensure you can get the sleep your brain, body, and baby need.

Tips for better sleep:

- Set up a bedtime routine for yourself and be consistent.
- Go to bed close to the same time every night and wake near the same time every morning.
- Stop stressful activities like watching the news, scrolling social media, or engaging in arguments 30 to 60 minutes before your desired sleep time.
- If you want something soothing prior to bed, try breathing exercises, guided meditation, gentle stretching, taking a warm bath, listening to calm music, or reading a paper book (not a digital one).
- Make your bedroom dark and quiet, and keep the temperature comfortable.
- Try not to drink alcohol or caffeine late or eat large meals close to bedtime.
- Physical activity during the day can help you sleep better at night.

Pregnancy and Panic

If you've had a panic attack before, then you know the feeling of worry or fear that can come with anticipating another one, especially the possibility of it coming at an inopportune time. For many people, panic attacks create their own anxiety about having a panic attack. If you're having more than an occasional panic attack and an ongoing fear for at least a month about having another attack or what will happen to you as a result of one, you may be experiencing panic disorder.

Some research suggests that prepregnancy symptoms can remain the same during pregnancy. For some people, symptoms of panic may lessen during pregnancy, while for others, panic may increase, potentially leading to postpartum depression.

Unfortunately, some of the symptoms of panic are also symptoms of pregnancy, such as nausea, shortness or shallowness of breath, sweating, heart rate changes, and occasional palpitations. If you're already vigilant about having a panic attack, some of the physical experiences of pregnancy can make you worry that you're having one. This intensification of anxiety is then another stressor on you and your body and potentially the baby.

Panic while pregnant can feel doubly difficult because of the worry that how you're feeling is affecting the baby. Your awareness of the life growing in you heightens your sense of responsibility and your levels of stress. This feeling of responsibility can also increase your vigilance of any symptoms you experience. Clients experiencing high anxiety during pregnancy often express their frustration that they are having panic at all and their worry of how it will affect the baby.

A client with panic might describe a scenario like this: Alex described feeling panic each time they went to the doctor's office for their checkup. Initially they didn't. However, after one doctor's appointment where their blood pressure was high due to a panic attack, they developed a fear of it happening again. Each time they went to the doctor, their heart felt like it was beating fast. When the doctor took their blood pressure, it was high, which made Alex more anxious. Alex's breathing felt shallower, they became sweaty, and then they grew more worried about the baby.

Let's take a closer look at your panic symptoms to try to differentiate, if possible, what is pregnancy anxiety and what is panic so that you can more clearly see what symptoms you can target for coping.

	SYMPTOMS OF PANIC BEFORE PREGNANCY	SYMPTOMS OF CONCERN IN PREGNANCY	SYMPTOMS THAT MAY BE DUE TO PREGNANCY, NOT PANIC
HEART RACING			
SWEATING			
TREMBLING OR SHAKING			
SENSATION OF CHOKING			
CHEST PAIN OR TIGHTNESS			
NAUSEA OR DIARRHEA			
DIZZINESS OR LIGHTHEADEDNESS			
FEELING LIKE THINGS ARE UNREAL			
NUMBNESS OR TIN-GLING IN HANDS OR FEET			
FEAR YOU MIGHT DIE			
FEELING LIKE YOU'RE LOSING CONTROL			
FEELING LIKE YOU'RE LOSING YOUR MIND			
HOT FLASHES OR CHILLS			

Unique to panic is that, in the intensity of the moment, you can feel like you're losing control or are going to have a heart attack or die. When you're pregnant, these feelings can be scarier because of the responsibility you feel for your baby. Stress management, relaxation skills, and breathing techniques are the go-tos for anxiety and panic management in general.

Identify Your Coping Skills

Often with panic and anxiety, people have coping skills that they forgot about, or they don't recognize the ways they are already coping. Here are some examples of possible coping skills when you feel panic and anxiety:

BREATHING TECHNIQUES: Slowing down your breathing, taking deeper breaths, box breathing, breath counting

THOUGHT MANAGEMENT: Reassuring yourself that you're okay, telling yourself that this will pass soon

PHYSICAL/BEHAVIORAL ACTIVITY: Walking, cleaning, stretching, yoga, running

GROUNDING OR RELAXATION TECHNIQUES: Mindfulness practice, meditation or guided meditation

Use the space below to identify what you're already doing to help cope with panic and anxiety:

BREATHING TECHNIQUES	THOUGHT MANAGEMENT	PHYSICAL/ BEHAVIORAL ACTIVITY	GROUNDING OR RELAXATION EXERCISES	OTHER WAYS YOU ARE MANAGING

Pregnancy and Obsessive-Compulsive Disorder

Alicia described an ongoing worry about a kidney problem that had started before pregnancy. She had medical testing that showed a very minor concern that was fixable with changes in diet. She was convinced that it was a bigger concern than the doctor said. She became pregnant shortly after, and she sought out advice from her OB-GYN, got a second opinion from a general physician, asked for as many tests as she could think of, scoured the internet for answers, and printed out information to show her doctor. She was convinced that her medical providers were either thinking she was anxious and minimizing her concerns or just telling her what she wanted to hear. Using regular coping techniques was extremely difficult because of her nearly constant need for reassurance from her therapist. Alicia was exhausted and overwhelmed from her worry, and it took up so much time in her day. She wanted it to stop but felt that it was out of her control.

Experiencing OCD during pregnancy is particularly difficult since there are many new situations that can trigger obsessive thoughts and compulsive behaviors if that is something you are prone to already. In addition, the responsibility of carrying a new life can bring feelings of great pressure. Although it is common to have some pregnancy-related worry, OCD can contribute to ongoing, persistent, and repetitive worry that feels hard to stop even with reassurance or self-soothing tactics. Stress also contributes to an increase in obsessions and compulsions during pregnancy.

IN UTERO FOCUS. Obsessions and compulsions in pregnancy tend to focus on the baby in utero, the health of the pregnancy in general, or the health of the carrier. Some research shows that the obsessions focus more on contamination and illness. Worry can be about needing things to be a certain way with the baby or pregnancy, the health of the baby in general, or the baby's movement or heart rate. Preexisting obsessions and compulsions can intensify during pregnancy as well, such as concerns about medical issues, body changes, orderliness, germs and cleanliness, sexual behaviors, or safety.

SOCIETAL AND CULTURAL PRESSURES. Another difficulty with OCD in pregnancy is the overlap of societal and cultural pressures related to pregnancy. The internal judgment of how you're "supposed to feel" during pregnancy can really run right up against many OCD symptoms. This is especially true for intrusive thoughts. For many people, intrusive thoughts in pregnancy can be more disturbing and upsetting, especially if the thoughts involve the baby in utero or postpartum. As stated before, this is anxiety for two (or more for multiples). Because the intrusive thoughts are unwanted, out of the blue, intense, and intruding on your mind, you can feel even more alarmed. One of the most common responses I hear is "What is wrong with me? I shouldn't have thoughts like that about my baby."

INTRUSIVE THOUGHTS. Unwanted, anxiety-producing thoughts will often bring up feelings of fear or disgust and can feel horrifying. A characteristic of these thoughts is that you do not want to have them, you do not want to act on them, and you feel appalled by them. This can lead to feelings of worry, shame, embarrassment, and a desire to keep them secret. It's important to remember that these thoughts are just thoughts and not intentions, nor do they carry any meaning about you as a person or parent. Other types of obsessive or intrusive thoughts can be related to the following:

- **Contamination:** Focusing on cleanliness, worrying about germs or illness affecting your health or the health of the baby
- **Sexual concerns:** Worrying about you or someone else having sexual thoughts, images, or motives about your child
- **Harm:** Worrying about something bad happening to the baby on accident or on purpose because of you or someone else

COMPULSIONS. Because the physical or mental acts of compulsions calm the obsessions, they can feel relieving at first. However, compulsions provide temporary relief and, in many ways, lend themselves to further obsessions. It's a reinforcing cycle that can feel very hard to stop. For instance, if you are obsessively worried about the baby's heartbeat, you may compulsively check it just to make sure. The feeling of the compulsion is that you must act on it. It feels like you have to check the heartbeat multiple times in order to relieve your worry. Compulsions can be mental acts as well, such as repeating a phrase over and over in your mind in response to an obsessive worry. These types of compulsions are repetitive, hard to stop, and excessive:

- **Checking:** Needing to look or feel many times to make sure that everything is okay with you or the baby
- **Safety:** Needing to hide or throw out sharp objects or anything that could cause harm or actively avoiding things that you fear could harm the baby
- **Mental acts:** Needing to repeat prayers, phrases, sayings, counting, or a mental act to relieve the obsession

REASSURANCE SEEKING. I see a lot of obsessive worry and reassurance-seeking compulsions in pregnancy. To be clear, wanting reassurance from medical providers, friends, and family is absolutely normal and fine. When the reassurance isn't enough and you feel the need to compulsively ask again and again if everything is okay, the need for reassurance becomes its own anxiety. But you are not your thoughts. The brain goes off due to stress and pressure. Your thoughts are thoughts. They do not define you.

DEPRESSION. Some people experience both OCD and depression during pregnancy and the postpartum period. People should be assessed for both. Personal and family history of depression can be one of the risk factors. However, in the general population, having OCD is a risk factor for depression. Having an anxiety disorder like OCD is exhausting for many people. An ongoing struggle of worry and stress can wear you down, especially if it feels like something you can't stop. This isn't necessarily the only cause of the depression, but it is a common one.

Exercises That Can Help

Exposure and response prevention (ERP) is often used in the treatment of OCD. This therapy is discussed a little more in chapter 4 and is best used with an ERP-trained provider.

Another strategy is the Schwartz four-step treatment method for OCD, which involves four essential steps to reduce the intensity of obsessions and compulsions. This method is useful over time to retrain your brain to not cause overwhelming thoughts and urges. This strategy helps you observe your thoughts rather than feel as if they are controlling you.

These are the four steps of the Schwartz method:

RELABEL. Notice your thoughts or urges and name them as what they are, thoughts and urges.

REATTRIBUTE. It's not because of you. It's because your brain is stressed.

REFOCUS. The thoughts and urges just happen. The power you have is in what you can choose to do with them.

REVALUE. The thoughts are going to come when they come, so accepting that they will come and that you don't have to take them seriously takes the air out of them.

Pregnancy and Post-traumatic Stress Disorder

One of the most amazing things about humans is their capacity for resilience. I see this so clearly in all of the perinatal clients who come in for therapy. People can know that they have had traumatic experiences but not know that the symptoms they experience are related to past trauma. Yet, here they are, still going, still pushing forward, doing their best in their day-to-day lives. Certainly, some people know that their history of traumatic experiences affects them, and they are actively concerned about how pregnancy will impact them.

Trauma is very personal. If an experience felt traumatic to you, then it was traumatizing, even if everyone around you says or thinks you're fine. Trauma, as they say, is in the eye of the beholder. Two people could go through the same exact situation and have very different internal experiences. One person might be shaken but feel generally okay, while the other person may be traumatized by it. No one can assume your experience for you.

People experience trauma in a variety of ways. You may have a clinical diagnosis of post-traumatic stress disorder (PTSD) or symptoms of trauma that do not constitute a specific diagnosis. Depending on the reason for PTSD, pregnancy can be a real trigger.

The prevalence of PTSD in the general population is relatively high, with rates being higher for women than for men. One of the ways PTSD can affect pregnancy is related to hormonal changes, especially higher levels of cortisol or the dysregulation of the body's stress response. Carrying a higher level of stress and being in a fight-or-flight mode often taxes your body.

Some people respond to trauma by numbing themselves or disconnecting from what happened or is happening to them. This is an adaptive response that occurs in the moment as well as in ongoing traumatizing situations. It's a form of mental, emotional, or physical survival. However, people can run into challenges with this form of coping as they can continue to experience numbing and disconnection when there isn't a trauma happening. In pregnancy, sometimes that can lead to feeling disconnected from the pregnancy, the baby, or physical sensations. It can also lead to avoiding certain memories, places, or people.

Past Trauma and Current Pregnancy

Trauma has a way of making your brain perceive that a situation that brought fear in your past will happen again. It can even make you feel like you're still there in the past when it happened, not just emotionally or mentally but physically as well. Your brain doesn't necessarily know the difference between an actual threat and an embodied memory, so you have to train it to know that the past is in the past and you are relatively safer now than you were at the time.

That said, if you're not in a safe situation, do not try to convince yourself that you are. You cannot self-care your way out of ongoing trauma. You can take care of yourself for sure, but trying to make yourself think that you should be able to handle an ongoing threat is not fair to yourself, nor is it reasonable.

Let's look at some ways that past trauma can show up in pregnancy.

RELATIONAL TRAUMA. If you had a difficult experience in your past with a primary caregiver or family member, pregnancy can bring up feelings that you had about them. Unattended or unhealed parts of your experience can potentially lead to fear or worry that you will be the kind of caregiver you had. (If you already have this awareness and are concerned about it and want to do better, you're already being a good parent.)

MEDICAL TRAUMA. This type of trauma involves a situation, procedure, medical provider, or place of treatment that felt traumatic to you. People have interactions with medical professionals at higher rates during pregnancy and the early postpartum period than at any other point in their lives, unless they are managing a previous medical condition. If you have a history of medical trauma, heading into the doctor or medical office for appointments or procedures can remind you of it.

RACIAL TRAUMA. Past experiences with medical systems where implicit bias or racism was at play in your medical care can bring up worry that you won't be believed or that your care won't be taken as seriously as it should be. Knowing that maternal mortality rates are higher for BIPOC can bring an additional level of traumatic stress due to heightened worry about your own experience.

PHYSICAL, MENTAL, AND EMOTIONAL TRAUMA. This type of trauma includes previous pregnancy loss at any stage, infertility challenges, past sexual trauma or physical assault, and accidents or losses of any kind that felt traumatizing to you.

Generally, traumatic experiences in pregnancy are related to these categories:

- Perceived or actual loss of control in decision-making regarding your body and birth wishes
- Perceived or experienced threat to your life or your baby's life
- Threats to you or your baby's physical integrity or safety

FINDING SAFETY

Pregnancy can be an intense time. Incidents of domestic violence and intimate partner violence can increase during pregnancy and put you and your baby at risk of harm. If you're in a relationship or situation where you are not safe, please look into these resources for support:

- National Coalition Against Domestic Violence: NCADV.org/resources. This resource page lists organizations and websites for many types of safety support, such homelessness and abuse.
- National Domestic Violence Hotline: 1-800-799-SAFE (7233)

Remember Your Resilience

You've come this far with all that you've been through. Even with all of the difficulties and concern you feel now, you're putting one foot in front of the other and making your way. The good news is that with the right help, support, and tools, you can heal even further and feel relief from these trauma symptoms. It can seem like you just have to live with what you've experienced or like healing feels too hard, scary, or impossible. I'm really glad to say that there are ways to feel better and ways to be able to heal enough to enjoy your pregnancy and baby.

I suggest the professional support of a therapist who has training in some form of trauma therapy. Some therapies to consider and research are eye movement desensitization and reprocessing (EMDR), somatic experiencing, trauma-focused cognitive behavioral therapy (CBT), cognitive processing therapy, and prolonged exposure therapy. In the meantime, revisit the list of PTSD symptoms in chapter 1 to see which ones are relevant to you.

It can feel overwhelming to think about these types of symptoms. Try to remember that you are here and not back in the past when those things happened. You got through all of that and are still moving forward, even if your thoughts and emotions feel stuck. This is resilience. You continue to keep going, and that says a lot about your strength and perseverance.

HIGHLY SENSITIVE PERSON AND ANXIETY

A highly sensitive person (HSP) is someone who feels things deeply, is often aware of how others are feeling, and has a high level of conscientiousness and awareness of subtleties in their environment. Anxiety is often a sign of or a side effect for people who have high sensitivity. Understanding this sensitivity trait can help you know why you feel the way you do instead of judging yourself for it.

There are a few traits that can show up during the perinatal period:

- Overwhelm/overstimulation
- Perfectionism
- Needing more down time or alone time
- Being more affected by other people's mood
- Being less likely to ask for help
- Being more intensely affected by sleep loss

To learn more about these traits and to see if you are highly sensitive, I encourage you to visit HSPerson.com and JulieBjelland.com to take a self-test. Elaine Aron's book *The Highly Sensitive Person* also has valuable information about HSPs.

Grounding Technique for Trauma

This technique is called five-senses grounding. It is useful for bringing you into the present moment as you use all of your senses, helping you get away from hypervigilance and distracting your brain so that it can get out of trauma land. It may seem simple. And it is, for a good reason. It's very hard to be engaged in complex thought when your brain is responding to trauma. Practicing a simple technique is easier so that you don't become more flooded or overwhelmed with another complex task.

Notice or list the following:

- 5 things you can see
- 4 things you can feel
- 3 things you can hear
- 2 things you can smell
- 1 thing you can taste

chapter three

Thought Modification

Stress and anxiety transform your normal thoughts into more abnormal thoughts, causing you to notice things through a negative lens or to carry irrational, fearful thoughts. In essence, this leaves you looking at a situation through a magnifying glass, noticing only a small part of the experience and leaving out many other details. Anxiety can find its way into even your most common, everyday thought processes, like making assumptions. It distorts how you perceive information and experiences and how you think of yourself and the world around you.

In this chapter, we will work on identifying, understanding, and managing those anxious, worried thoughts as they are specifically related to pregnancy.

How to Change the Dialogue

It's possible to not even realize that your thoughts are negative or that they are affecting how you feel. The thoughts can be so frequent and normal that you might not even notice you are having them. One of the first and most effective ways to change a pattern is to be aware of it. Once you can identify your thought patterns and negative thoughts, then you can decide what to do with them.

The fight-flight-freeze nature of the anxiety response affects how you perceive and think about a situation, whether the stress is physically in front of you or a possible bad outcome in the future.

Identifying and Labeling Your Thoughts

Let's first identify some of the most common thought distortions that therapists see and hear in clients who are pregnant or trying to get pregnant. Thought distortions are when your thoughts become negative, rigid, and inaccurate. As you read through this section, you may notice that you engage in many of the distortions discussed. Please note, this is not another thing to be anxious about. Everyone has thought distortions. They're pretty common, especially when situations are new or unclear. However, if you have anxiety, thought distortions can create a greater amount of distress and further perpetuate your anxiety.

Identifying Negative Thoughts

Read through each of the negative thought distortion examples. If the thought distortion applies to you, write how your own thoughts are similar or different.

EMOTIONAL REASONING. This distortion leads you to think that if you feel something, it must be true. During the transition into parenthood feelings can frequently get mistaken for facts, especially if you're feeling vulnerable and anxious.

- **"I am alone."** I feel lonely; therefore, I am alone. No one cares.
- **"I feel like a bad mom."** I feel bad; therefore, I must be bad.

  My emotional reasoning thoughts:

  _____

  _____

ALL OR NOTHING. This thinking assumes that thoughts are black or white, good or bad.. This process of thinking excludes the context of the situation and leaves no room for any gray area.

- **"I'm already a bad mom."** I can't see the ways that I am a good mom.
- **"I'm a failure because I can't get my anxiety under control."** I can't control my feelings, so I'm bad.

  My all-or-nothing thoughts:

  _____

  _____

  _____

CONTINUED ▸

Identifying Negative Thoughts continued

OVERGENERALIZING. This is a thought process where how you perceive one situation becomes how you think every future situation will turn out. You can overgeneralize about your own experiences or what you observe from other people.

- **"I always mess up."** One mistake or difficulty makes me feel like I will always make mistakes.
- **"I'll never connect to my child."** Feeling disconnected in pregnancy brings fear that I'll never connect.

My overgeneralizing thoughts:

_____

_____

WHAT IF? This is a method of questioning the future that feels negative and doesn't actually get answered. If a question stays a what-if in your mind, it contributes to fear, worry, and anxiety.

- **"What if I can't get to the hospital on time?"** Then something bad will happen.
- **"What if my partner doesn't help?"** Then I'll be all on my own.

My what-if thoughts:

_____

_____

CATASTROPHIC THINKING. When something relatively minor happens, you see it as horrible or the worst possible outcome. This high anxiety usually leads you to thinking about the worst-case scenario.

- **"I can't drive because if I have a panic attack in the car, I won't know what to do or how to get help."** One worried feeling leads to the worst fear.
- **"If I have gestational diabetes, my baby will be unhealthy or unwell, and it will be all my fault."** You think a diagnosis means that you've done something wrong.

My catastrophizing thoughts:

_____

_____

DISQUALIFYING THE POSITIVE. Good things that happen don't count because it feels like you got lucky or someone else made it happen. Sometimes this includes a double standard, where you can see the positive for other people but not for yourself.

- **"People are only being nice because I'm pregnant."** It doesn't seem like people can be nice just to be nice.
- **"They only came by to help because they feel obligated."** You can't see that people want to support you.

My disqualifying-the-positive thoughts:

_____

_____

CONTINUED ▸

Identifying Negative Thoughts continued

JUMPING TO CONCLUSIONS. Without any experience or evidence, you are sure of something and make assumptions or predictions about how things will be.

- **"I just know I'm going to mess my baby up."** There is no evidence. You haven't messed anything up, but you feel sure that you will.
- **"The birth is going to be horrible."** There is no issue that would indicate a bad birth, but fear makes you think there will be a bad outcome.

  My jumping-to-conclusions thoughts:

  _____

  _____

"SHOULD" THINKING. These are inflexible ideas or rules about how things should or shouldn't be. When the should is directed at yourself, you can feel shame or guilt. If the should is directed at someone else, you can feel frustration or anger.

- **"I should be happy I'm pregnant."** You feel pressure to be or feel a certain way.
- **"They should know what I need. It's clear that I'm tired."** You feel resentment or anger that others aren't caring for you.

  My should and shouldn't thoughts:

  _____

  _____

MENTAL FILTERING. This is when you focus only on a negative part of a situation. All of the positives get reduced or go unnoticed. Even if there is some truth to a fear or a negative situation, it's not the whole picture.

- Your coworker sends you a note of encouragement, but there's one comment that feels negative, and you focus on that all day.
- Your friends host a baby shower for you, but one friend didn't come because of a misunderstanding, and that's all you can think about.

My filtering thoughts:

_____

_____

PERSONALIZATION. This occurs when you attribute something to yourself that is actually unrelated to you or your actions. You may hold yourself accountable for things that have nothing to do with you or are out of your actual control.

- **"My friend didn't call me back yet; she must be mad at me."** There may be many reasons why your friend didn't call.
- **"It feels like there is a problem, and it must be my fault."** Even if there is a problem, there are many different things that could have caused it.

My personalization thoughts:

_____

_____

Your Brand of Negative Thoughts

There are many types of cognitive distortions and many ways that anxiety can impact your thinking during your pregnancy journey. If the ones listed in the previous exercise don't quite resonate with you, there may be other ways in which your thoughts turn negative or become distorted. Think for a moment on the thoughts that you notice most often that are connected to stress, anxiety, fear, or worry. List them below so that in the future you can more easily notice when they are coming.

Strategies for Changing the Way You Think

Now that you've expanded your awareness of ways that your thoughts may be unhelpful, it's time to learn some options for managing those thoughts. First, we will look at what contributes to stressed thinking, both on global and individual levels, and identify the stressors that contribute to anxious thoughts. Then, we'll break down ways to cope and manage. In doing so, you can move from automatic negative thoughts to an intentional redirection of your thoughts that fosters nonjudgmental awareness and change.

Global or Environmental Sources of Anxiety or Stress

Global, societal, cultural, and local issues absolutely affect you and your stress load. Consider 2020, a year marked by a global pandemic, civil unrest, collective trauma, global and local political issues, natural disasters, restrictions on day-to-day activity, and massive changes in the way people work and go to school. The impact of this stress on you personally will wax and wane, but it's still ever present. It has an impact on hopeful and new parents in ways that can be hard to put into words. Fears of what your child will be born into, how to get the perinatal care you and the child will need, what the birthing environment will be like, and what kind of supports or supplies will be available to you. Anxiety becomes so personalized during pregnancy, so it's important to recognize and remember that environmental stress can increase your anxiety. Looking at stress from this perspective is meant to help you remember that it's not just you.

Systems of Influence

▼

The following diagram illustrates Bronfenbrenner's ecological systems theory. Its purpose is to show how our different environments, situations, and life contexts influence each other and, therefore, negatively and positively affect us as individuals. We are always in the context of our lives; however, in Western cultures, the individual tends to be viewed as the one who's responsible for how things turn out. But there are always other influences and forces that are acting for us and against us. By stepping back from your solo experience and taking in the complexity of your context, you can gain some perspective as to why you may be feeling stressed or anxious.

Use the circles in the diagram to think about what your stressors and supports are in the context of your life right now. For each circle, think of the factors that may be affecting you or that you may be affecting in a positive, negative, or neutral way. By having a deeper understanding of the systems of influence, you can step away from blaming yourself for things being difficult and see how the other factors may be affecting you.

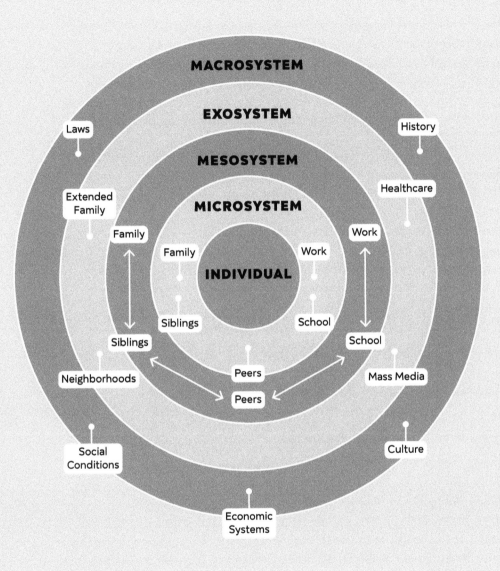

Macrosystem: Culture and society
Exosystem: Influenced indirectly
Mesosystem: Relationships between microsystems
Microsystem: Immediate environments

Implicit Messages about Pregnancy and Parenthood

Some of your deepest and most strongly held beliefs about yourself and who you are in the world drive your thoughts, feelings, and behaviors. Digging a little deeper into your belief system can be tough, but it's a necessary journey. Some of your beliefs come from societal messages or cultural norms about pregnancy, having a baby, and parenthood. These types of beliefs can take the form of collective myths about what motherhood, fatherhood, or parenthood is supposed to be like.

Other beliefs come from the families that you grew up with and how they define what a good parent is. These beliefs can be hard to identify, in part because they can be so integrated into how you see yourself or your role as a new parent.

You can start to identify your beliefs or the myths that you've learned along the way by asking yourself what you believe you're supposed to do, be, or think about pregnancy and parenthood. One other way to identify these beliefs is to notice if you're labeling what you do or think with a value judgment of "good" or "bad."

These are some of the most common myths or beliefs:

- *I'm supposed to be happy to be pregnant.*
- *I'm a bad parent. I should be grateful.*
- *A good parent is supposed to be with the baby all of the time.*

Day-to-Day Sources of Anxiety

Your basic needs are so often overlooked that it's easy to forget how they might be affecting you. Before going into detail about these anxious thoughts, it's important to remember that other sources of stress or strain may be contributing to how you feel. You get into routines and patterns that become so regular that you don't notice your fundamental needs are being ignored. I hear so often that people don't eat until midday or evening because they didn't have time. Then they wonder why they are tired or don't feel right. Sometimes the answer is to adjust your routines to allow for fundamental self-care.

Even though these are day-to-day needs, they affect how you feel and think. This is especially true during pregnancy, when you may feel more tired, be more or less hungry, and have increased energy demands on your body and mind. Being attentive to your needs can ease the intensity of other stressors, increase your capacity to cope, and support your sense of safety and connection.

Banishing Bad

▼

List the ideas or beliefs you carry with you about what "good" parents and "bad" parents are supposed to do, feel, or think. Then ask yourself if this is a belief you want to keep and why, giving special attention to how the belief impacts your anxiety.

	GOOD PARENT	BAD PARENT	KEEP?	WHY OR WHY NOT?
THOUGHTS				
ACTIONS				
FEELINGS				
BEHAVIOR				

Back to the Basics

▼

How often are you making sure that you have enough water, food, rest, or interaction with other people? Your busy life can keep you from noticing health and wellness factors. Look through the following list and reflect on what you regularly ignore and what you might need more of in your life.

Fundamental questions to ask yourself:

- *When was the last time I ate? Am I hungry?*
- *Have I had any water or other fluids today?*
- *Have I been getting enough sleep? How many days in a row has my sleep been disrupted?*
- *Does my body want or need exercise or gentle movement?*
- *Do I have any health conditions that are contributing to how I'm feeling?*
- *Is there any medication that I take regularly? Have I taken it today?*
- *Have I had any increased stress from work, home, relationships, or life in general?*
- *Do I feel safe in my home and work environments?*
- *Do I need or want supportive contact with others? A hug? A conversation?*

Based on this list, what do you need to attend to or ask for support with? Get familiar with this list of questions so that when you can't quite tell how you're feeling, you can ask yourself the questions and quickly assess what your needs are.

Identifying Your Individual Anxiety and Stress

At the beginning of any anxiety response, there's a stressor, which is the thing that creates stress for you. If we were to trace back from your anxious thought to the situation that caused the anxious thought, we would probably find the stressor. There are thoughts that just pop in out of nowhere, but sometimes even those have a source. When you're aware of the context of your life, the things that contribute to your anxiety, you can more easily identify the reason for it, rather than just feel flawed that you feel anxious. Pregnancy itself may be one of the main stressors you're dealing with; however, other life stress can also increase pregnancy anxiety.

Identifying Your Thoughts and Feelings When They Are Happening

Sam has an ultrasound scheduled and has started to worry about the growth of the baby. The last ultrasound was fine. The doctor didn't have any concerns. However, Sam's mind starts to go over everything she's eaten and how much she's exercised over the last month. Sam worries because the nausea with pregnancy has made it hard to eat much. Thinking about the upcoming ultrasound, she starts to feel tightness in her chest, and her mind begins to race. Sam feels antsy and starts to notice all of the things in the house that need to be cleaned up, so she begins cleaning, feeling a bit frantic, like she can't sit down. She starts to feel overwhelmed and flustered because she can't remember what she was going to do next.

Being aware of your thoughts and feelings, or at the very least having a process for identifying them as they happen, can help prevent your anxiety from spiraling out of control. It may seem simple to just notice, label, and identify the thoughts and feelings, but it's hard to make a change if you don't know what's happening.

Name That Stress

▼

Take a few minutes to write down your current life stressors, relationship challenges, or situations that are creating or contributing to your stress. Once you identify what your stressors are, you can discern if they are something you can work through or wait to deal with them at a later time.

_____

_____

_____

_____

_____

_____

Having said that, take what you've learned so far and consider the example of Sam. When you read the example, are you able to identify what is happening? Consider taking time to reflect on your own anxiety process and identify what is happening. The more often that you take time to do so, the more familiar you will become with your patterns and be able to identify where you can cope.

Stopping the Anxiety Cycle

When a stressful thing happens and you are in a state of anxiety, it can prompt a cycle that can feel out of control. Sometimes this happens so quickly that you can't even pinpoint what stressful thing started it all. If you take a moment to slow the cycle down, you might be able to see how to manage it.

The stressor starts the cycle and quickly puts thoughts, feelings, physical responses, and behaviors into action. Consider the previous example of Sam, and let's look at her anxiety in the form of a stress wheel.

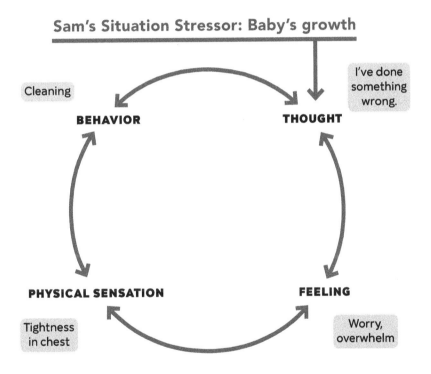

Sam's Situation Stressor: Baby's growth

Give Yourself a Choice

Anxiety can really make you feel like you're stuck or don't have a choice. It can feel hard to stop. Like a wheel, the anxiety seems to just keep rolling along. But you are learning ways to apply the brakes. Based on what you have learned so far, where are there possibilities to intervene or stop the spinning?

- Consider the stress wheel and the nature of its repetition.
- Look at the thought log provided, and list your stressors or triggers.
- Next, list the negative thoughts you notice.
- What are your emotional, physical, or behavioral responses to this stress?
- Consider an alternative response, and make a note of it.
- What are other ways that you could think in this situation?

Offering yourself an alternative can really help remind you that you have options when you're in the midst of an anxiety response.

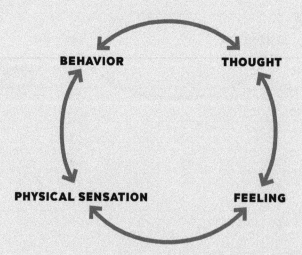

BEHAVIOR   THOUGHT

PHYSICAL SENSATION   FEELING

Thought Log: Alternative Thoughts

STRESS/ SITUATION/ TRIGGER	AUTOMATIC NEGATIVE THOUGHT	RESPONSE (EMOTIONAL, BEHAVIORAL, PHYSICAL)	ALTERNATIVE RESPONSE
Baby's growth.	I've done something wrong.	Worry, chest tightness, cleaning	The doctor said the baby was healthy and fine, so it's possible that the baby is still growing well. My belly is a little bigger than last time.

Treat Yourself as You Would Treat Others

Imagine that your best friend is going through the exact same thing you're going through. They come to you and tell you what's going on and that they are anxious, worried, sad, or stressed out about their pregnancy. Then you tell them, "Just get over it. All you have to do is think positively. What's wrong with you? You should be happy you're pregnant." How do you think they might respond to you? Alarmed, angry, or offended? You better believe it!

But when you are feeling the same things and you talk to yourself that way, it seems justified, right? Why is it okay to talk to yourself that way but not to your best friend? This is important to think about. When your thoughts have space and time to fester in your mind, they take on a life of their own. Then you begin to feel bad about yourself, and you aren't even sure why. It's often because of the negative voice (your own) that has been berating you all day. It's no wonder you feel bad.

What You Consume Becomes Your Thoughts

Each day, you are inundated with news, social media, magazine covers, radio programs, and a number of other informational sources. This barrage can feel overstimulating and can increase anxiety and stress. You have a ton of information at your fingertips that you can easily access at any hour of the day. The downside to this availability particularly affects pregnant people with anxiety or trauma. Anxiety, obsessive-compulsive disorder (OCD), and trauma make you want answers to questions, and pregnancy brings up a lot of questions that want answering. So, searching the internet for "how to tell if my pregnancy is going well" brings up answers to that question along with 10 new questions to research. Sometimes the information you find can trigger or contribute to more anxiety and worry.

Social media is a beast of its own when it comes to anxiety and making people feel bad about themselves. The online portrayal of perfection can make it seem like everyone else has it together. If you are like most people, when you experience stress and anxiety, you tend to compare your worst self to everyone else's best self. That leaves you feeling worse. A rule of thumb: If you start to feel agitated, anxious, or down while scrolling online, it's past time to stop scrolling.

Internet Stress

▼

What have you noticed that contributes to you feeling anxious when you're online or browsing social media? If you haven't noticed how you feel yet, this is a great time to reflect on how you are affected by your time online. One common feeling is angst or agitation, especially if you spend a lot of time online and definitely if you're reading stressful material. It can almost feel like the internet is pulling you in, even when you want to pull away. You may even have data from your phone that tells you how much time you spend in each app. People often spend more time than they think.

For this exercise, either check your phone stats or give as good an estimate as you can about how much time you spend in each area, how it makes you feel, and what you could or would like to do instead.

	HOW MUCH TIME DAILY?	HOW DOES IT MAKE YOU FEEL?	WHAT COULD YOU DO INSTEAD?
SOCIAL APPS			
NEWS			
INTERNET SEARCHING			

After looking this over, how do you feel? This exercise is meant to help you think about what you want for your time. There is no judgment, no right or wrong, just observations so that you can see if the internet is contributing to your stress.

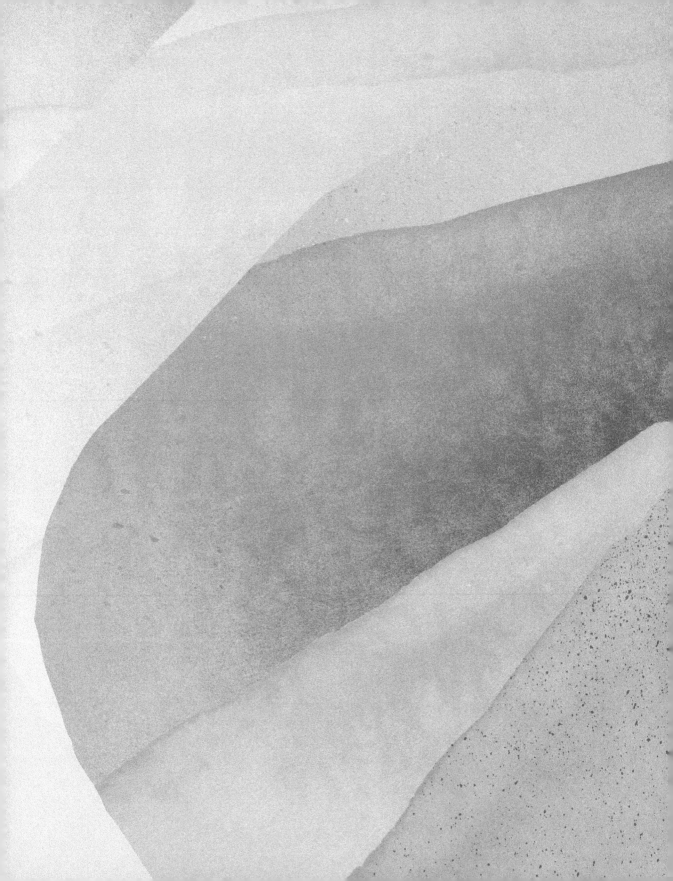

chapter four

Managing Distressing Thoughts

In my work with perinatal clients and in my personal experience as well, distressing, upsetting, and scary thoughts are the hardest to experience and hardest to talk about with someone else. They can feel shameful, embarrassing, or unlike you. Many people describe the need to keep these thoughts hidden from others, which in turn also makes them feel worse about the thoughts. Silence and secrecy regarding your emotional pain can make you feel isolated and alone. It doesn't have to be that way. It is important to highlight that distressing thoughts are common with different types of anxiety, stress, and trauma.

Unwanted Anxious Thoughts

Having distressing, scary, and unwanted thoughts is more common than you may know. Since not many people talk about them, it might seem like you're the only one experiencing them. Feeling like you have to keep unwanted thoughts to yourself actually increases anxiety. People question themselves about why they have these thoughts. They feel guilt and shame, and they feel alone and stuck with their distress. Specifically, during pregnancy or the postpartum period, there is a lot of pressure to act as if you're fine and happy. So, when anxiety-producing thoughts show up, it's even more difficult to understand why they are there, which is all the more reason to know that these types of thoughts are not just in your head and that you can talk about your stresses with other people.

Intrusive Thoughts

Intrusive thoughts are unwanted thoughts that pop into your head. They can come seemingly out of nowhere or be related to a situation you are in or something you are thinking about. The thoughts are often about something bad happening to you or someone else. They can include a visual of the thought or be accompanied by a physical or visceral negative response, like a "yucky" feeling. These types of thoughts can feel overwhelming, embarrassing, shameful, and even terrifying.

You don't need to have a diagnosed mental health condition to experience an intrusive thought. They are relatively common in the general population. Your brain sometimes creates random or strange thoughts or connections to unrelated things. Generally, if one of these thoughts pops into your mind, you can just brush it off, even if the thought was a bit distressing. But if it sticks around or is becoming repetitive and causing more distress, then it could be a sign or symptom of a mental health condition.

If anxiety, obsessive-compulsive disorder (OCD), panic, or post-traumatic stress disorder (PTSD) are a part of what you're dealing with, intrusive thoughts are even more distressing. The unwanted thoughts can contribute to or create their own anxiety about why they are there. You may feel confused as to why you are having them and what they mean, and you may be very anxious about the possibility that you will act on the thoughts, even though you know that you never would. You are not alone in experiencing such thoughts or in trying to unthink or reshape the thoughts.

Noticing Distressing Thoughts

▼

Are you experiencing any thoughts that pop into your mind and feel random or unexpected?

_____

_____

_____

Are the thoughts distressing, scary, or embarrassing? Do they bring up feelings of fear or shame?

_____

_____

_____

Do the thoughts come and go, or do they stick around for a while?

_____

_____

_____

If they stick around, how do you cope?

_____

_____

_____

Intrusive Obsessive-Compulsive Disorder Thoughts

Anya came to therapy at about six months pregnant with high anxiety, convinced that there was something wrong with her baby that the doctors just couldn't see. She'd gone to the OB-GYN multiple times and asked for every kind of test that she could imagine, and the doctors honored all of her requests. All the tests came back confirming that Anya and her baby were medically clear and that the baby was developing at a healthy rate. Then Anya read online about a symptom that she didn't know about before. She felt sure that she had that symptom and needed to go to the ER right away to have it checked. She was medically cleared; however, because her heart rate and blood pressure were high, the doctors suggested psychotherapy and a medication for anxiety. In her therapy session, Anya stated that she was so tired of being worried, she felt exhausted by her mind, and her partner was getting frustrated with her. She said, "I'm sure I sound crazy." Anya listed all of her concerns and then asked her therapist if they thought she had the condition she was worried about. Her therapist consulted with her OB-GYN to get their perspective. It became clear that Anya was seeking reassurance from any and all providers, but the reassurance was never enough to quell her worries.

The intrusive thoughts associated with OCD during pregnancy are repetitive, distressing, and unwanted. Although there are several types of intrusive thoughts, during pregnancy, they tend to center more on illness or contamination. Other thoughts can be related to harm coming to the baby or pregnancy, distressing thoughts that are sexual in nature, thoughts of immorality, or thoughts that make you doubt yourself or your actions. There is a slight increased risk for development of OCD in pregnancy, in part because the sense of responsibility for protecting this new life is heightened, especially for first-time parents.

As you read through this section, remember, thoughts do not equal desire, intent, or action. Just because you have a thought does not mean you're going to act on it. People who have intrusive distressing thoughts are alarmed by them, sometimes even horrified that they had the thought in the first place. This experience can lead to the person questioning themselves, wondering why they would have such a horrible thought or what is wrong with them.

In actuality, when people have intrusive thoughts and OCD, they do everything they can to not engage in the feared thought. Compulsions manifest for this exact reason: to make sure that nothing bad happens. The thoughts feel like an imminent or intense fear, and the actions feel like the antidote. I like to think that OCD in the perinatal period is a person's sense of responsibility and vigilance that comes from a place of love but is turned up so high that it becomes fear. Taking your responsibility for a new life seriously puts your mind into hyperdrive as it looks out for any possible signs of harm. Because of all this, shame is a very common experience with OCD and intrusive thoughts, and the shame often leads to secrecy.

In OCD specifically, there are obsessions and compulsions that may be thought related. A person with a clinical diagnosis of OCD recognizes that the obsessions and compulsions are unreasonable, irrational, or excessive. They do not want to be experiencing this and are trying everything they can not to. The compulsions take time away from other things in their lives and are distressing in and of themselves. In the example, Anya's obsession was worry about illness. Anya's compulsion was to seek reassurance. She felt burdened by this concern and knew that it was irrational, but she couldn't stop worrying.

Obsessions and Compulsions

Let's look more at ways that obsessions and compulsions may present themselves. This is not an exhaustive list.

Obsessions

Obsessions have four components:

1. Persistent and recurrent thoughts, images, or impulses that are intrusive, inappropriate, and distressing.

2. These thoughts aren't just big worries about actual problems.

3. The person tries to ignore the thoughts or suppress them with some other action or thought.

4. The person knows that the thoughts are from their own mind.

Most common types of obsessions (preoccupation, excessive and/or illogical thoughts) center on these concerns:

ILLNESS OR CONTAMINATION: Obsessions with cleanliness or germs, worry that something you ate will affect the baby, worry that something you touched was germ-ridden

HARM: Worry that you or someone else will hurt the baby on accident or on purpose, violent or graphic images of harm to you or someone else, worry you will act on an impulse to harm yourself or someone else

DOUBT: Doubt about decisions you've made, worry about the baby's heartbeat or vitality

SEXUAL: Distressing thoughts of sexually abusive behaviors toward the baby

Noticing Obsessions

Do you notice any of these components or types of obsessions in your mind? If you experience obsessions, they may not be included on this list, but they are still valid.

What type of obsessions do you experience?

Compulsions

Compulsions can be behaviors or mental acts and can be identified by the following:

1. The person feels compelled to do the compulsion in response to the obsession, or the person feels compelled to follow a rigid set of rules.

2. The goal of the compulsion is to reduce anxiety, stress, or dread of the obsession. The compulsive acts are excessive, and they may or may not be specifically connected to the obsession itself.

Types of compulsions:

REASSURANCE SEEKING: Repeatedly asking your family, friends, or medical providers what they think about your concern

CHECKING: Checking for your baby's heartbeat, checking the internet for answers, checking your body

CLEANING: Washing your hands repeatedly, sanitizing or sterilizing things you or the baby may touch, cleaning your home often

AVOIDANCE: Avoiding sharp objects, things that may be contaminated, being alone, being in certain places or with certain people

MENTAL ACT: Some type of mental act in your head, such as prayer, counting, or another action that makes the obsession reduce in intensity

ORDER: Focusing on symmetry, exactness, perfection, or alignment of objects

Noticing Compulsions

Do you notice any of these components or types of compulsions in your life? If you experience compulsions, they may not be included on this list, but they are still valid.

What type of compulsions do you experience?

_____

_____

_____

_____

_____

_____

_____

_____

_____

EXPOSURE AND RESPONSE PREVENTION

Exposure and response prevention (ERP) is a type of cognitive behavioral therapy that is frequently used to help manage OCD. In the exposure part of ERP, the therapist helps the patient take inventory of their obsessions and rate their subjective level of distress to those fears and obsessions. Then the therapist slowly reduces the patient's level of distress by exposing them to their fears, starting with the least intense parts, and couples this exposure with relaxation techniques to lower the intensity of the fear. The patient continues working their way up to the more intense fears until they feel like they can cope with those, too. The response prevention supports the patient in their desire to stop engaging in compulsive behaviors. Compulsions temporarily help reduce anxiety, but they also become part of what keeps the anxiety going. It is common to feel anxious about this type of therapy because it sounds like you're getting rid of the thing that helps manage the anxiety. But actually, you're learning new ways to cope that reduce your anxiety and increase your ability to manage overwhelm. It is important to seek out a psychotherapist trained in ERP for this type of therapy work.

Identifying Other Types of Scary Thoughts in Pregnancy

There are several mental health conditions that, when more severe, can result in difficult, scary thoughts. There are some intense thoughts listed here, so gauge for yourself whether you can read through them. The goal is to be able to identify whether you have any of the types that feel unmanageable. If so, it is worthwhile to look into professional support.

PANIC. This includes frightening, panicked thoughts, such as "I'm going to die," "I'm going to have a heart attack," "I'm losing my mind," "I'm out of control," or "This is never going to end."

PTSD. This involves recurrent, intrusive, and distressing memories, thoughts, images, or perceptions about a traumatizing event from your past. People who experience PTSD will avoid thoughts related to the trauma. They often worry that something bad will happen, and have difficulty believing things will be okay.

DEPRESSION. Hopeless and helpless thoughts can manifest when symptoms are more severe. These thoughts can include thoughts of wanting to just leave and drive away, thoughts about death or not wanting to be alive anymore, thoughts that your baby would be better off without you, thoughts about doing something harmful to yourself, or thoughts about suicide.

RAGE. Feelings of rage can come with anxiety and depression. They are often overwhelming, intense, and scary for the person experiencing them. You can have sensations of anger that make you feel like punching walls, hitting your partner, or taking other aggressive actions that can also be related to your pregnancy or baby.

PSYCHOSIS. These are delusional thoughts that would sound bizarre to someone else. Psychosis can also manifest as hallucinations, hearing voices, deep confusion, great difficulty tracking time, disorientation to place or time, being highly agitated, or not sleeping much or at all.

OCD AND PSYCHOSIS

OCD and psychosis are not the same thing. The scary thoughts that come with OCD can be distinguished from the ones that come with psychosis by how you experience them. With OCD thoughts, you will want to avoid them, have compulsions to stop them, not want to accept them, and have anxiety and worry because of them. You will do everything you can to not engage in the behavior you're worried about. People with OCD are considered at no risk or at very low risk of harming themselves or someone else.

With psychosis, depending on how quickly it develops, there may be a period of confusion in which the person worries about how they are feeling. They may feel off or like they can't hold on to their mind. However, the behaviors and thinking process break from reality and become delusional (believing something that's not real) or hallucinatory (seeing or hearing things that are not there). The person will accept the delusional thoughts as truth, and other people cannot convince them that the thoughts are not true. Psychosis is a medical emergency. People experiencing it are at a high risk of harm to themselves, to someone else, or to the baby.

Identifying and Labeling Your Scary Thoughts

In many ways, you experience your own thoughts in the first person; you are the narrator of your inner mental life. You become accustomed to your own way of thinking and believing about yourself and the world. When it comes to anxious, stressed, and traumatic thoughts, you naturally assume that those thoughts need to be listened to. Therefore, you experience your thoughts. One way to manage this overwhelm is to become an observer of your thoughts rather than a participant in them. Being an observer allows you to have a little perspective, identify what's happening, and label the thoughts in a new way.

Anxious Thoughts Are Thoughts, Not Actions

One reason intrusive thoughts feel overwhelming is because of what your brain does to try to make meaning of them. Often people are worried that if they had an aggressive or distressing thought, they might act on it. A key factor in managing these types of thoughts is to recognize that they are just thoughts, with no basis of evidence. Ask yourself:

- Is the anxious thought something you want to have happen?
- Is there evidence that your thoughts make things happen?

Anxious Thoughts Do Not Define You

Anxiety, OCD, PTSD, panic, depression, and other conditions can feel very personal, even more so when you're on the road to parenthood. These conditions turn your thoughts negative. "What's wrong with me?" is a question I often hear from pregnant and postpartum people. It's crucial to understand that mental health conditions are something you are going through; they do not make you who you are. Ask yourself "What am I going through?" instead of "What's wrong with me?" Observe your thoughts instead of judging them. A thought does not define you. A thought does not carry a covert meaning about you.

- Are you your thoughts?
- Do your thoughts actually dictate or define who you are?
- Is there evidence for the judgmental reaction to the thought?
- Is there a different way to observe the thought?

Anxious Thoughts Happen, but Acceptance Helps

"Just stop thinking about it" sounds like nice advice, but if you've ever tried it, you know it doesn't work. Suppressing or ignoring our thoughts doesn't make them go away. Pushing thoughts away can feel necessary when they're upsetting. However, this strategy backfires in the long run when it comes to coping with big feelings like worry and fear.

Thoughts and feelings that are pushed away are actually still there. They're funny that way. They need to be expressed to a certain extent, or they will just fester and grow until they come out in a more intense way like anger, panic, or resentment. Also, focusing on not thinking about something actually makes you think about it.

Distinguishing between Acceptance and Resignation

Accepting your thoughts doesn't mean that you want them or like them. You're just simply acknowledging their existence. Being resigned to the thoughts, on the other hand, is feeling that the thoughts will always be there, that there's nothing you can do about it, and that you are powerless. Resigning yourself to your thoughts isn't supportive as a thought management strategy.

Other Anxiety and Stress Management Techniques: Distraction

Short-term, temporary distraction is very useful. Helpful distraction entails intentionally turning your attention to something else to help stop the cycle of anxiety, rumination, or distress. This type of redirection does not need to be complex. You don't need to specifically search for a positive distraction. You can choose something neutral or not emotionally charged.

Examples of healthy distraction include grounding techniques, playing a game (word search puzzle, sudoku, matching games, etc.), using mindfulness, calling a friend, going on a walk, turning on soothing music, or counting backward by fives.

Thought Experiment

What you're focused on is what you see. Have you ever had the experience of wanting to purchase something specific like a certain brand of shoes and then you start to notice people wearing them everywhere you go? This same phenomenon happens with negative unwanted thoughts. If there is something you don't want to think about and you tell yourself not to think about it, you'll think about it. This is because you're focusing on not wanting the thought. Try this exercise:

1. Don't think about a cup of coffee.

- What's in your mind now? A cup of coffee?
- Stop thinking about coffee.
- Can you do it? No, because you're focused on that coffee now.

2. Now try this:

- Okay, cup of coffee. I see you. Fine, you're there. I'd rather not think about you, but there you are.
- I'm going to think about tea now. I love peppermint tea.

Can you feel the difference in the two ways of thinking in this little experiment? The first part is a fight. It's you versus coffee. Coffee wins because it's the focus. The second part is acceptance. Coffee is there. You don't have to like coffee. You don't have to be friends. It just is. You win because you don't have to fight.

Distraction Is Not Avoidance

Avoidance is often used as a way to cope. However, avoidance isn't great for long-term coping as it tends to be maladaptive over time. If you find that you are avoiding a feeling, thought, or situation, you may also feel tension, worry, anxiety, or fear. You'll have to assess for yourself whether safety is a factor. If it is, please seek safety. However, if there is space to cope in a different way, then addressing the thing you're avoiding can actually help reduce the stress.

Taking Time to Worry

Worry can take over so much of your day. When there aren't many distractions, your mind may start to wander and worry. Or upon waking, your brain can be worrying about anything and everything. Worry pops in whenever it wants and might even disrupt a perfectly good period of work or rest.

Consider this example of how worry works:

1. *What is this pain in my side?*

2. *I hope the baby is okay.*

3. *If I ask my doctor, they are going to think I'm that anxious pregnant person who wonders about everything.*

4. *Maybe it's nothing. But what if it's not?*

5. *I'll look up my symptom online.*

6. *Well, it looks like it could just be ligament pain. What if it's gallstones?*

7. *What are the symptoms of gallstones? I'll look them up.*

8. *Okay, I don't have a fever, but this feels weird.*

9. *Maybe it will just go away if it's ligament pain.*

10. *Okay, I'm going to try to sleep.*

11. *What in the world is this pain in my side?*

To combat your worry spiraling out of control, you can schedule "worry time" for yourself. It may seem counterintuitive to schedule time to worry, but doing so can establish some parameters for your anxious mind.

Worry Time

▼

1. Schedule a time every day where you can spend about 20 minutes with your worries. Try to schedule it at least two hours before going to sleep. You don't want to worry too much before bed. Ideally don't schedule it for when you wake up either, as you don't want to start your day off with worry.

2. During your designated worry time, write down all of your worries. Be sure to include all the worries that you can think of, all the worries that you've saved up throughout the day or night, and really let yourself get in there and worry. You don't need to solve all of the worries, but writing them down may solve some of them along the way.

3. Look into each worry. Try to remember why it came up or what started it.

4. Redirect worries at other times of the day to your scheduled worry time. When you notice your mind wandering off in worry, gently stop and tell yourself that you will attend to that worry during the scheduled time.

This practice takes time, patience, and a bit of awareness building to notice when worry is happening. If you're concerned that you won't remember a specific worry, you can jot it down. Being able to reflect on and distance ourselves from our worry can also help us get perspective. It is possible that a specific worry warrants further attention. It is also possible that after reflecting, you can see that the worry was temporary or just seemed really big at the time.

Answering What-Ifs

Think about all of the times you've asked yourself, "What if?" More often than not, a what-if is a worry about something bad happening in the future. How many times have you actually answered your what-if? When these questions go unanswered, they linger, the anxiety and tension grow, and the worry gets deeper. But what if you could take the air out of the balloon of worry by following your what-if to its logical end? You can! You can take the worry out of it by asking, "Then what?"

- *What if my parents won't help take care of the baby when it gets here?*

  → *Okay, what if? Then what?*

- *Then I'll have to find another childcare option.*

  → *Okay, then what?*

- *Then I'll have to interview nannies or day cares.*

  → *Okay, then what?*

- *I guess I'll figure it out when I need to.*

Important Notes on Working through Anxiety

Anxiety and fear can make any task feel impossible. Have you ever thought of something that you needed to do and felt so overwhelmed that you didn't do anything? If you have, then you know your anxiety about the task grows, making it feel even harder to do. Then, the task doesn't get done, and the guilt sets in. So, when it feels like too much, how do you move forward? Start with something small. Find a skill or exercise that feels a little challenging but still doable. Just do that one thing. Once you've been able to do that, do the next task that feels slightly difficult but still beneficial. The idea is that you do one task and allow yourself to feel some sense of accomplishment. Then the next task might feel easier to approach. You can use this tool throughout pregnancy and postpartum as well. One step at a time gets you where you want to go.

What-Ifs

▼

In this exercise, you can reduce the anxiety associated with an unanswered what-if by using logical conclusions.

   List each what-if below, then follow the "then what" process until you get to a logical, possible resolution. Notice if your worry is emotionally based, and if it is, try to think of what a logical conclusion might be. This exercise isn't meant to discount your concerns. Rather, it is meant to help you temper high emotionality with some grounded logical possibilities.

WHAT IF?	THEN WHAT?	THEN WHAT?	THEN WHAT?	THEN WHAT?	CONCLUSION OR POSSIBLE RESOLUTION

chapter five

Relaxation Techniques

Relaxing in the face of anxiety, post-traumatic stress disorder (PTSD), obsessive-compulsive disorder (OCD), or panic can feel challenging. Relaxation techniques take practice and time to learn and integrate. While it's difficult to start something new in the middle of fear, worry, and trauma responses, practicing when you're not very anxious can make it easier to use these techniques when you really need to. Relaxation techniques can also be a way of taking care of yourself and your baby at the same time. Reducing stress in your body is a benefit to your baby as well.

As you embark on trying new relaxation techniques, please know that not all techniques work well for all people. Some of them may work better for you than others. If you can, try each one out for several days to see if you feel any benefit. If a technique doesn't work for you, that's fine. Try another. If you have a history of trauma or any triggers that are related to a relaxation practice, it's okay to modify it in a way that helps you feel safe, or you can just not use that technique. The goal is to help you relax, so be aware of any increase in worry or anxiety. If it's tolerable and you want to continue, go ahead. If it's not tolerable, then move on to something else.

Breathing

Breath regulation is one of the most reliable relaxation exercises because your breath is always with you. You don't need any special tools or special training, and you can use this technique at any place at any time. You're doing it right now. Simply bringing a level of awareness to your breath can have a positive impact and helps you notice what your natural breathing pattern is. As you regulate your breath, you regulate your blood pressure, heart rate, stress response, and mental responses, and all of that benefits your pregnant body and your baby. Deeper and slower breathing can help reduce anxiety and the tension in your body for both of you.

tip

If you feel lightheaded at any time while practicing a breathing technique, you should stop and resume your normal breathing. If you're new to regulating your breath for relaxation, it can take a little practice to feel comfortable.

Diaphragmatic Breathing

Diaphragmatic breathing, also known as belly breathing, is the practice of breathing deeply in and out of your belly, expanding your diaphragm while keeping your chest relaxed. The diaphragm is a muscle at the base of the chest; it separates your chest from your abdomen. Breathing in expands the diaphragm and breathing out relaxes it. Deep breathing pulls in air to as much of the lungs as possible. Anxiety often creates a shallow breath that feels more like breathing in and out of your chest. Regulating your breath is the simplest and most straightforward way to manage anxiety. Taking deeper, slower breaths signals to your brain that it's okay to relax now.

One of the challenges to deep breathing in pregnancy is that the baby is taking up space as they grow, which can make breathing a little shallower. Taking a deep breath at eight to nine months pregnant is very different from taking a deep breath at two to three months pregnant. If you find that very deep breaths are hard, just breathe as deeply as you comfortably can.

Diaphragmatic Breathing

▼

The diaphragm is a muscle at the base of the chest under the lungs that separates the chest from the abdomen. For this exercise, you'll use the full capacity of the diaphragm to pull as much air into the lungs as possible, then allow it to slowly release back to the resting point.

1. Sit comfortably or lie down. You can keep your eyes open or closed, whichever feels more comfortable.

2. Put one hand on your belly and the other hand on your chest. If you cannot use your hands for this exercise, bring your attention to your belly and chest.

3. Breathe in through your nose, down into your belly to the very base of your lungs, expanding your diaphragm and filling your abdomen as much as possible.

4. Notice that your belly expands or rises as you breathe in.

5. Keep your chest rested and still.

6. After you've taken in the deepest breath you can, let it out slowly through your mouth or nose as your diaphragm returns to its resting point.

When you exhale, don't force more air out than is natural. This type of deep breathing can feel a little uncomfortable or awkward, especially if you are used to shallow breathing from your chest. Start with three breaths in and out, then over time work your way up to a timed practice of two to five minutes twice a day. You can use diaphragmatic breathing whenever you want to calm your body and mind.

Square Breathing

Square breathing, also called box breathing or four-square breathing, can help with stress reduction and concentration. It consists of slowly breathing in, holding the breath in, slowly breathing out, and holding the breath out.

Breath Counting

This type of breathing uses counting as you inhale and counting as you exhale to pace your breath. Breath counting can help you regulate your breathing rate and focus on your breath and counting instead of anxiety and worry.

Guided Imagery

Guided imagery is a type of meditation that uses your mind, imagination, and other sensory experiences to take you on a gentle, pleasant getaway and help you find calm. Your mind is very powerful. With some suggestion through visualization, you can recall a place that brings you peace and happiness or make up an imaginary place that's just yours. You can use this mental imagery and mental space anytime you want or need calm. This place is always available to you because it lives within you, just as your breath does.

Visiting this peaceful, familiar, or special place in your mind helps you rest mentally, physically, and emotionally, giving you a break from anxiety. One of the benefits of this type of relaxation is that you don't have to think too much. You just have to allow your mind and body to experience the calm that comes with being gently guided along.

There are many guided meditations to help you connect with your pregnancy and baby, manage your anxiety during pregnancy, and get ready for labor and delivery. Thankfully, with technology, there is no shortage of places to find guided meditations.

Square Breathing

This exercise is a way to regulate your breath while having mindful focus on counting. The process of taking slow, measured deep breaths helps manage stress.

1. Sit in a comfortable position. Keep your gaze soft, or close your eyes if you are comfortable doing so.

2. Breathe in through your nose for a count of four.

3. Hold the breath in for a count of four.

4. Breathe out through your mouth for a count of four.

5. Hold the breath out for a count of four.

You can assess for yourself if a count of three, five, six, or more suits you best. Try three cycles of breathing. Then over time, work your way up to a couple of minutes twice a day. You can use this technique whenever needed.

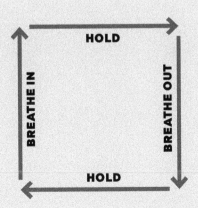

Breath Counting

▼

Breath counting enables you to use your mind and body together to reduce stress by distracting you and focusing your attention on your breathing.

1. Sit in a comfortable position. Keep your gaze soft, or close your eyes if you are comfortable doing so.

2. Breathe in to a count of four.

3. Breathe out to a count of four.

Depending on how comfortable you are, you can decrease or increase the count of four to a number that feels manageable.

As you're starting out, try to do this exercise three times. Then as you get more comfortable, expand to three to five minutes twice a day. As with any breathing exercise, you can practice at any time and implement the breathing whenever needed.

Guided Imagery

▼

For this practice, it's helpful to listen to someone guiding you. This is just an example of what guided meditation can be like. You can follow along and see what it might feel like for you. You, or someone else who has a voice you find soothing, can record this guided meditation so you can listen to it as often as you'd like.

1. Sit or lie down in a supported position that is comfortable for you in a quiet space with the lights low. Take a couple of moments to just notice your breath in its natural rhythm.

2. Soften your gaze, or close your eyes if you feel comfortable doing so. Now, take an intentional deep breath, slowly filling your lungs with air. Breathe out slowly. Again, take a slow deep breath in. Release that breath. Notice your body relaxing as you release the breath.

3. Let your mind wander to a place high in the mountains. Allow yourself to experience the different sensations—the sun shining and gently warming your skin, a cool, crisp breeze floating to you with the clean smell of mountain air, the sound of the breeze gently blowing through the trees. This place has a calming energy with the strength of the trees and the stability of the mountain. Feel the ground holding you as you stand on this mountain.

4. You start to walk on a well-worn path that meanders toward a meadow. Along this path, you see lush green grasses. You notice small purple and yellow wildflowers nestled in patches throughout the grass. In the distance, you hear the gentle trickle of water. As you look into the distance, you notice butterflies and dragonflies fluttering in and out of the grasses. You naturally take a breath and feel more relaxed as you take in your surroundings. A slight smile

CONTINUED ▸

Guided Imagery continued

comes to the corners of your mouth, and a sense of peace touches your heart.

5. Continuing to walk toward this meadow, you find yourself feeling more deeply connected to nature and the land you are on. Your breathing feels easy, your body feels relaxed, and your mind feels light. The sound of water is getting closer with each step you take. After several more steps, you come to a clearing and a beautiful meadow that looks out to another mountain range in the distance. The sound of water becomes clearer, and you see a small stream that has cut through the grasses. The water is crystal clear and nurtures the grasses and the life in the meadow. The path you're on weaves through the meadow, gradually upward at a slight incline, crossing the stream several times. Taking your time, you walk through the clearing, noticing the trees that line the meadow and the calm you feel as you see that the butterflies and dragonflies are now joined by hummingbirds and are all dancing together.

6. You see a couple of boulders at the end of the path that look like a perfect place for sitting. As you approach them, you see that the source of this stream is a freshwater spring coming directly out of the mountain. The water is cold and plentiful, a constant, steady flow of the purest water. Cupping your hands, you gather some water and taste the best water you've ever had—sweet, ice-cold, and energizing.

7. After a few sips, you take a seat on the rock next to the spring. Feeling the warmth of the sun, with your eyes closed, you ask yourself if you will find the healing you are seeking. Just then a breeze comes through the meadow toward you, bringing a felt sense of peace and a knowing that everything will be okay. The feeling of contentment you have brings peace to your whole body. You feel relaxed, calm, and centered.

8. Take several breaths in your natural rhythm and just be.

Progressive Relaxation

Progressive muscle relaxation (PMR) is the process of tensing and tightening each muscle or muscle group one by one, then releasing that muscle tension into relaxation. This practice is useful for reducing stress and anxiety and for supporting sleep. Another benefit of this exercise is that it allows you to tune in to how your body feels when it's tense and when it's relaxed. With anxiety, you often hold tension in your body without even knowing it. The tension itself partly contributes to anxiety because physical tension signals to the brain that there is stress, and the brain when stressed will signal to your body to tense up and get ready for anxiety. Practicing PMR retrains your muscles to relax and helps you tune in to the difference. The more aware you are of your body's patterns, the better able you will be to manage the stress response. As with any new relaxation practice, you'll need to practice PMR regularly for the best benefits.

Specifically, if you're experiencing anxiety conditions in pregnancy, PMR helps relax your body, benefiting both you and your baby, and it can help you prepare for birth and the postpartum period. As your body shifts and changes in pregnancy, you may have muscle tension in new places or increased tension in places where you have a habit of holding it. Relaxing those muscles can help with your overall comfort during pregnancy. In addition, having less tension in your body can help with the birthing process and the overall stress response in labor. In the postpartum period, relaxing muscle tension can be very helpful. Babies can co-regulate to a certain degree with you, so it helps when you and your body are in a calm state. PMR can also support your physical well-being because holding a baby, feeding them, and changing them can be a strain on your muscles. Learning to see where you're holding tension or feeling tight can help you care for your own body as you're caring for your baby. If you are having difficulty falling asleep, try PMR before bed as part of a bedtime routine to help ease you into sleep.

Progressive Muscle Relaxation

This relaxation practice allows the mind and body to work together to release muscle tension and emotional stress. Some of its benefits can be noticed immediately, while others come over time with repeated practice. Try to allow for consistent practice over several days to see how it helps you be aware of and release tension in your body.

As you go through the exercise and each muscle group, tighten the muscles for five to seven seconds, then release and relax them for about 20 seconds before moving on to the next muscle group. When you're relaxing, try to notice how different it feels for those muscles to be relaxed. You can start at your feet and move up your body, or you can start at your head and move down your body. Try to practice for 10 to 15 minutes a day.

1. Find a quiet place to sit or lie down. You can keep your eyes open or closed, whichever is comfortable for you. Take a couple of deep, slow breaths to settle yourself. Notice where you have tension in your body.

2. Starting at the top of your head, tense the muscles in your scalp and forehead. Release your head muscles. Notice the relaxation.

3. Next, tense the muscles in your face, purse your lips, squint your eyes, and tighten your jaw. Release your facial muscles and jaw. Notice the relaxation.

4. Now, tense the muscles all around your neck and throat. Release them. Notice the relaxation.

5. Shrug and tense your shoulders and upper back. Release the muscles. Notice the relaxation.

6. Flex your biceps and upper arms. Notice the tension, then release the muscles and feel the relaxation.

7. Tighten your fists and forearm muscles, then release and relax them.

8. Come back to your chest. Tighten it, then release it.

9. Pull in your abdomen, tightening as much as possible depending on your comfort level in pregnancy. Release and feel the relaxation.

10. Squeeze your buttocks and hips, feel the tension, then release and feel the relaxation.

11. Flex your quads as tight as you can, then release them and notice the relaxation.

12. Flex your calves and lower legs, hold, then release them into relaxation.

13. Curl your toes and tense up your feet. Release them and feel the relaxation.

14. Take several minutes to stay in your relaxed state. Breathe deeply and notice if you've tensed up again anywhere. If you have, release those muscles back into relaxation.

Additional Relaxation Practices

Anxiety management and relaxation practices are readily available in many forms, several at no financial cost. Some techniques are so common that we may not think of them when listing what we do to take care of ourselves. When you're anxious and pregnant, anything that works to help manage how you're feeling is great. If you're experiencing anxiety, it can feel like doing simple self-care isn't enough, but rest assured, it all counts. All of the following practices can greatly benefit your health and well-being.

PRENATAL YOGA. Thousands of years old, yoga has historically been a deeply spiritual practice. Only in modern times has it become a more physical practice related to relaxation, strength building, and stress relief. It's now widely practiced across the world and easily accessible on the internet. There are many studies that show the benefits of yoga, including stress relief, reductions in preterm labor, decreased pregnancy discomfort, and other benefits for both the pregnant person and the baby. One review of research showed that yoga in pregnancy is safe and can decrease symptoms of stress, anxiety, depression, and pain. The review also noted that yoga can increase emotional well-being and immunity in the pregnant person. Depending on the type of yoga or the instructor, you may be connecting to not only yourself but also your baby in utero. Sometimes people cry during or after yoga, and that's okay. It's often a sign of releasing feelings or stress.

During pregnancy, prenatal yoga, gentle yoga, or restorative yoga are the safest options, but talk with your medical care provider before engaging in any exercise programs.

WALKING OR EXERCISE. Gentle movement or exercise that you can do safely can change your headspace for the better. It can have calming or mood-boosting effects that can help your brain and body regulate more easily. Regular exercise also helps with sleep by decreasing your overall stress levels. It can decrease symptoms of anxiety and depression as well. Pregnancy can sometimes require limiting the intensity or frequency of your exercise or movement in general, so be sure to check with your medical provider to make sure it is safe for you.

GETTING OUTSIDE. Being away from your home and out in the fresh air can give you a change of environment, a change in perspective, and a positive distraction. Changing your environment by going outside really helps get your mind out of thought patterns you feel stuck in. It's like your brain needs something new to respond to in order to get it out of the spiral of worry. As you breathe in the fresh air, look around at nature or other city environments. Just not looking at a pile of dishes, for instance, can give you a break, even if for a moment. Don't underestimate the power of a couple of moments of intentional peaceful distraction. They might be just enough to help shift where your mind is for the day.

REST. You might not be surprised to hear that resting is hard for someone who has anxiety, panic, OCD, or PTSD. I often hear clients talk about the list of things that need to get done or the difficulty they have with resting because they feel fidgety, worried, or like they need to be productive. Sometimes the hardest thing to do is to allow yourself to rest guilt-free. Your body is busy growing a human, so your rest is productive. Rest is also an act of radical self-care in our modern society, which is too busy and focused on productivity. Rest isn't lazy, selfish, or something to feel guilty about.

MUSIC. Putting on some of your favorite music can shift your mind just enough to have some moments of feeling good. You can even make a feel-good playlist for yourself and turn it on when you need to change your energy. If you can get a little body movement in there, too, that would help even more.

OTHER FORMS OF RELAXATION. Many types of stress-relieving services are available. With the support of your care team, consider self-care options like prenatal massage, pregnancy chiropractic care, acupuncture, craniosacral therapy, or somatic therapies.

---

tip

Reduce your caffeine intake, especially at nighttime. Caffeine can increase your sense of anxiety because it is a stimulant and affects your central nervous system.

When trying these practices, remember that if it works for you, it works. If it doesn't work for you, it doesn't work. People can get caught up in thinking that all of these practices should work, and if one doesn't, then they think that they're doing something wrong. Try to be mindful and present with the process to see what works for you.

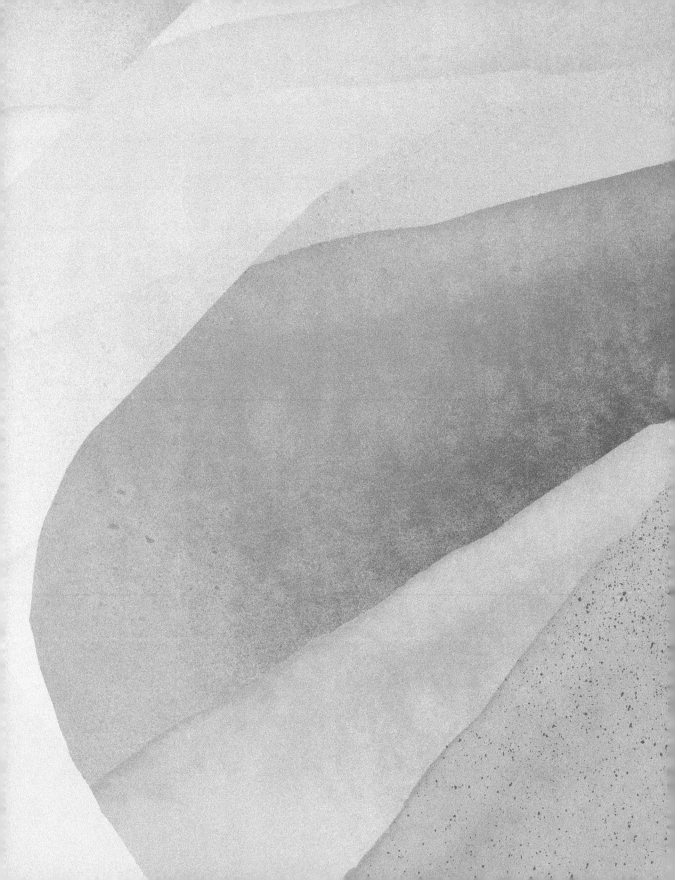

chapter six

Mindfulness and Meditation

Mindfulness and meditation are known to have a positive, healing effect on the mind and body. These practices can reduce anxiety and lower stress, depression, and physical discomfort during pregnancy. Other potential benefits are reduced inflammation, lower blood pressure, and increased attention, awareness, and insight. Although mindfulness and meditation have expanded beyond their roots in Eastern spirituality into a modern therapeutic practice, their advantages have been known for centuries, and they have been employed by doctors and patients for just as long. Mindfulness and meditation are closely related and overlap in many ways; however, there is a distinction between them.

Mindfulness

Mindfulness is a state of being in the present moment, noticing and paying attention to what is happening within or around you without judging it. You can engage in mindfulness anywhere at any time, and you can be mindful about anything. You can use mindfulness in meditation. You can use it for any daily activity, no matter how simple or mundane, like brushing your teeth, cleaning, eating, or driving. For instance, when you're brushing your teeth, where are your thoughts usually? Are you thinking about your day, what you need to do next, or a conversation you just had? You're probably not paying attention to what you're doing. When using mindfulness, you are not doing anything else but brushing your teeth, noticing everything you can about the experience. This helps you be in the moment, slow down your mind, have awareness of your body, and practice directing your awareness to the present moment. Mindfulness can help with regulating emotions and reducing stress in pregnancy.

Many skills, tools, and techniques that we've already discussed in this book use mindfulness:

- Wise mind
- Awareness and labeling of cognitive distortions
- Self-reflection
- Schwartz treatment method for obsessive-compulsive disorder (OCD)

- Five-senses grounding exercise
- Worry time
- Breathing exercises
- Guided imagery
- Progressive muscle relaxation

Meditation

Meditation uses a variety of techniques to train the mind to focus, increase awareness, manage stress, and calm the mind and body. It also helps you observe your mind. You can use meditation to ease anxiety by slowing down your mind so that it is aware instead of vigilant. Anxiety is a state of fear and worry about the future, and meditation is a path to bringing yourself out of that anxiety and into the here and now. Meditation does this by using your mind-body connection to send signals that you are safer than your anxiety is leading you to believe. There are many types of meditation and many ways to meditate. Some variations of meditation practices use mantras, movement such as walking, or a focus on the breath. They can be guided or unguided, spiritual or secular.

Pregnancy Mindfulness and Meditation

When you're pregnant or trying to become pregnant, your awareness is expanding to include the life of the baby developing in your belly or of the baby you want. You may notice your body, mind, and emotions in a new way as well. Becoming a parent is a life transition that presents people with mostly new-to-you experiences. You are in the process of learning, making changes, and quite possibly relating to yourself and others around you in new ways. With all of this change, it's understandable that anxiety can increase.

Using mindfulness and meditation during pregnancy can be helpful to reduce anxiety, manage stress, connect to the pregnancy or the baby, and connect to your body. There are limited studies on the effects of mindfulness, meditation, and yoga on pregnancy, but most demonstrate positive benefits for both the pregnant person and the baby. Specifically, they show some reduction in anxiety, depression, and pain symptoms when the technique is practiced for several weeks. It's worth pursuing an ongoing practice to see how it can benefit you.

You can tailor your mindfulness and meditation practice to include visualizing a healthy baby and pregnancy, bringing calm to the baby and pregnancy, supporting connection to your baby, being in tune with and accepting your body changes, feeling more at ease with any condition you are managing, being more open to accepting the unknown, and feeling connected to yourself as you transition into parenthood.

Common Barriers to Using Mindfulness and Meditation

Although mindfulness and meditation practices can have such positive effects, some people can still be hesitant to adopt these practices. Being mindful or meditating can cause you to notice thoughts, feelings, emotions, or physical sensations that you'd rather not be aware of because they are uncomfortable, intense, or worrisome. The goal of these practices is to pay attention, to check in with yourself, and to become aware. The awareness part is key. Without awareness, it is harder to address your anxiety, which can allow it to run free, forcing you to respond and react rather than manage and resolve the feeling. Bringing your thoughts, feelings, and sensations into awareness is a powerful tool for managing anxiety.

One issue I hear a lot from clients is that they don't meditate because they say that meditation doesn't work for them. They may have tried it a couple of times and didn't see the benefit. To be clear, not every technique works for everybody; however, it can require time and practice to really feel the benefits of meditation. Very few tools work well the first couple of times we try them. Meditation is a practice that takes practice. Retraining your brain to focus its attention where you are directing it is an ongoing effort. It can be frustrating to have to keep at it, especially if you feel overwhelmed and anxious. There's no magic number of times or length of time to try a new method of stress management, but giving it a good effort over a couple of weeks can make it feel easier.

Another common misconception about meditation is that it means not thinking about anything at all. Some people who try meditation for the first time feel that since they can't turn their brain off, they aren't doing meditation correctly. The reality is, your mind is always thinking. You can't stop it. Our brains are constantly processing most things around us and whatever we have in our direct attention. They're always taking in information from our surroundings, sensing, processing physical and environmental cues, and listening and getting information from our bodies. Most of what our minds and bodies perceive happens without our conscious awareness. Can you imagine how overloaded you would feel if you were fully aware and in tune with everything at once? Every sound, physical sensation, visual stimulus, smell, taste, thought, feeling, and interaction? It would be so overwhelming that you couldn't function. Basically, you can't not think, but you can redirect your mind.

When we are dealing with anxiety, OCD, panic, or trauma, attending to our minds can be overwhelming. There are some very good reasons that someone would turn away from conscious awareness and just try to get through what is going on. A person can feel flooded emotionally, and their mind can become hyperfocused and magnify fearful things or jump from worry to worry or become foggy. If this is what happens for you, simply take note of that without judging the experience. There is no right or wrong here. The goal is to just notice and have that awareness.

There are many culture-specific modalities for centering and connecting to the mind-body that use techniques like mindfulness, ancestral connections, prayer, spiritual healing, and rites of passage into parenthood. If you belong to a culture that uses these practices, it may be useful to look into supportive practices in pregnancy that align with your way of understanding the transition to parenthood.

If you are just starting out in a practice of mindfulness and meditation, you can start small with two minutes twice a day. Work your way up to five minutes twice a day, then to 20 to 30 minutes at each session. The goal is to build the skill on a regular basis so your mind is attuned to relaxation and can more easily navigate there when stress arises.

MINDFULNESS, MEDITATION, AND PREGNANCY LOSS

For those who have experienced pregnancy loss, mindfully connecting to a baby in utero can be overwhelming at first, especially if they haven't been able to grieve or experience some healing after the loss. Many parents who've lost a baby describe hesitating to connect to the current pregnancy or avoiding connection altogether because they fear another loss. Staying disconnected from the baby may be a method of protecting yourself from further pain, but each person's experience is different. Practices that include visualizing your baby or talking with the baby could be difficult, or they could be healing. In addition, people often feel angry or disconnected from their own body after a loss and even in a subsequent pregnancy. When engaging in mindfulness and meditation during pregnancy, it's helpful to be aware of your triggers and take note of what contributes to your sense of anxiety. If you can use mindfulness and meditation to connect to your body and baby, it can be incredibly supportive and healing.

Practices for Calming Your Mind, Body, and Emotions

Mindfulness practices aren't just for the mind; they are for the benefit of your whole self. These practices can include any and all of your senses, they can be related to an activity you are doing, and they can be done in physical stillness or any combination that works for you. The goal is to be present in whatever it is you are doing. Anxiety and stress can take our minds elsewhere and prevent us from experiencing what we are actually doing. By doing activities mindfully and intentionally, we can reduce our anxiety and potentially extract more contentment from each activity.

MINDFUL COLORING. Coloring for adults has become an increasingly popular form of mindfulness practice. Giving your full attention to choosing colors, coloring, and creating beauty and calm are the main goals of mindful coloring. You can find many varieties of coloring books to purchase as well as free downloadable coloring pages online. There are also many different styles of art to color. Some people love symmetry and patterns. Other people like to color pictures of nature, human figures, or animals. When coloring, be with the colors, be on the page, and notice your intentions and desires about coloring. When you are coloring one part, focus on that part. If you find that your mind is moving on to another part, redirect your mind to notice what you are coloring. There is no right or wrong in coloring. Just notice what your mind wants to do and do that. Use those moments to stay focused on coloring, and when your mind wanders, bring it back to the art and creativity of coloring.

OTHER ARTS AND CRAFTS. If coloring isn't exactly what soothes you, look for other art-based activities that allow you to focus, notice, and be present. Some ideas are painting, knitting or crocheting, drawing, making things with fabric, crafting, hand lettering, origami, making a collage, working with clay, sculpting, or anything else that brings calm and focus.

SITTING MEDITATION. Find a quiet and comfortable place to sit. Sit upright in a position that is supportive. If you are able to sit cross-legged or in lotus position, you may do so. As you sit, notice if you want to leave your eyes open with a soft gaze or if you prefer to close them. As you settle into your supported position, take one deep cleansing breath, then breathe at your normal rate for a moment. Notice any areas of tension in your body, then release that tension and settle a bit more. If you notice any distracting elements of your environment, just let them go and settle a bit more deeply.

The focus for this meditation is your breath. Notice the sensation of the air entering your nose as you inhale and exiting your nose as you exhale. Notice the rise and fall of your belly and chest. Inhale and exhale while settling more into your supported position. Anytime your mind wanders to other thoughts, topics, worries, or sensations, notice them without judgment and return your attention to your breath. Your mind may wander again. That's okay. If you notice any sounds from your environment, return your focus to your breath and notice it. Inhale. Exhale. As your mind wanders away from your breathing, notice your thoughts as they come up, such as concerns about the baby, a doctor's visit, or your health. Let these concerns float away. You may have some uncomfortable or painful thoughts and feelings. Gently acknowledge them, then let them fall to the wayside again. It's okay if it takes a moment or two. Just continue to redirect your awareness to your breath, the rise and fall of your belly, the sensation of the cool air entering as you inhale and the warmer air exiting as you exhale. Continue breathing and returning your focus to your breath as distractions come.

Mindfulness with Difficult Emotions

You are an emotional being. And yet somewhere along the way, you have likely been taught to push away feelings, ignore them, and think of them as a sign of weakness. Feelings and emotions aren't inherently bad or negative. Rather, they just are. Your feelings are a signal to you that you are having a response to something.

If you've ever tried to ignore a feeling, then you know that it will stay despite your best efforts. It just comes out more intensely some other time. Acknowledging and being aware of emotions lets them pass by and reduce in intensity. Because many cultures overemphasize keeping emotions in check, a lot of people who go to therapy might not be aware of their feelings, or they may be hesitant to experience their feelings because they fear the feelings will take over.

I've talked to people time and time again who come in for therapy with feelings that overwhelm them, but they do not know why. As we talk through their situations, part of the work is to identify and name the feelings. As soon as we identify the feeling or I ask something like, "Do you feel scared?" the tears come. We have discovered a fear or worry that they hadn't yet been able to put into words. The awareness and acknowledgment bring a release, and the crying reduces the intensity of the feelings. This is the ebb and flow of emotions. Emotions are like the weather. They come and go, but they don't stay for long.

Follow these steps to practice mindfulness with your difficult emotions:

1. Notice the emotion.

2. Turn toward the emotion. Allow it to be there.

3. Accept that the emotion is there. Embrace it with care, as an observer.

4. Understand that the emotion won't be there forever. You can allow release as it passes through.

The process of mindfulness has been described by Buddhist monk Thich Nhat Hanh in *No Mud, No Lotus* as how an in-tune parent responds to a child's tears. The parent sees the sadness of the child, scoops them up in an embrace, does not judge them, and gives them care and validation. The child then feels soothed and relieved. This is what you can do for yourself with your emotionally mindful practice.

Mindfulness and Visualization with Difficult Thoughts

As we've discussed, thoughts happen. Sometimes a thought is disturbing or upsetting, especially if it relates to worry about your pregnancy, your body, or the baby. When we take these thoughts seriously and try to get meaning out of them, we often get wound up in the angst of why we had the thought in the first place or what it says about us. One way to disengage from this spiral is to use mindfulness. Becoming an observer of your thoughts rather than a participant in them can help you see the thought as a thought and nothing else. Think about it. If a stranger says something rude or ridiculous to you, it's easy to blow it off because there's no personal connection. If you said that same thing to yourself, you might take it seriously. When it's not personal, it's just an observation and easier to let go.

Here's one way you can practice mindfulness and visualization with your difficult thoughts:

1. Notice the thought. See that it is there. Know that it is just a thought.

2. Imagine a beautiful flowing river. Visualize fall leaves resting on top of the water, slowly floating by. This river is here to support you in releasing your thoughts.

3. Place each difficult thought on a leaf and see the flow of water take it away.

4. Allow these difficult thoughts to leave you, knowing they are fleeting and temporary.

5. With each thought you place on a leaf, take a deep breath in through your nose and release it with a sigh from your mouth.

6. Know that if those thoughts return, you can place them on another leaf at any time.

Body Scan Meditation

Your body holds you, allowing you to experience the world around and within you. A body scan is a slow process of intentionally noticing each part of your body, one area at a time. A full body scan meditation can take 30 to 45 minutes for deep relaxation. If you need to, you can modify this exercise to a shorter time such as 5 to 10 minutes and still bring mindful awareness to your body. The anchor for this meditation is breath and body awareness. You notice any sensations, emotions, or thoughts that arise as you bring awareness to each part of your body. Some things you may notice include physical and emotional sensations, temperature, tingling, pain, release, pressure, tension, no feeling, or softness. Whatever shows up in your awareness is okay. Being aware and paying attention to the signals from your body can help you release what you need to. Any thoughts or feelings that come up may have significance, and you can acknowledge them as a part of the process.

Body Scan

▼

The purpose of a body scan is to mindfully tune into your body, allowing any thoughts or sensations to pass by without judgment, and focus on feeling present, calm, and connected to your body. Moving from your feet all the way up to your head, focusing on each part of your body for about a minute, you'll bring awareness to how your body feels to better notice and resolve any feelings of tension, pain, or discomfort.

1. Find a safe and comfortable space to lie on your back, or on your left side if that is more comfortable at your current stage of pregnancy. You can also sit if you'd like.

2. Taking a deep breath, bring your attention to your right foot. Notice any sensations that are in, on, or around your foot. Breathe here for a minute with focused attention on your foot, acknowledging and allowing any sensations you experience.

3. Now bring your attention to your right calf. Then move it to your right knee. Then focus on your right thigh and hamstring. Next, move your attention to your right hip.

4. Focus now on your left foot, then your left calf, your left knee, your left thigh and hamstring, and finally, your left hip.

5. Now focus on your pelvis and buttocks. Next, move your attention to your lower back. Then focus on your lower abdomen.

6. Continue moving through the middle parts of your body: your middle back, your middle abdomen, your upper abdomen, your chest and upper back, and your shoulders. Be sure to give each part focused attention.

7. Now begin to scan your right upper arm, moving down to your right forearm, then to your right hand.

8. Next, bring your attention to your left upper arm. Then focus on your left forearm and then your left hand.

9. Move your attention to the top parts of your body: your head, neck, face, forehead, and scalp. Be sure to give each part focused attention.

10. Now bring your attention to your body as a whole, noticing the integration and connection of all of your parts. Be with this feeling while continuing your deep breathing for a couple of minutes.

11. Slowly bring your attention back to your surroundings, take a cleansing breath, and notice any change in how you feel overall.

Walking Meditation

You often get from point A to point B without conscious awareness of how you got there. This happens in part because you have so many other things on your mind that take you away from what you are doing. Walking meditation lets you experience walking in a deeper, more reflective way, and it helps you develop embodied awareness while calming your mind. This type of meditation can be a soothing way to keep movement in your day if it's medically safe for you to do so. Focusing on the mental and physical aspects of walking is a great way to practice mindfulness, regulate your breathing, and be in touch with your body. This practice can be helpful throughout pregnancy, especially as your belly grows or you become more uncomfortable, and it's a nice way to stay connected to your body in a positive way.

Walking Meditation

You can do this type of meditation anywhere at any time. You can wear shoes or go barefoot depending on where you prefer to walk. This is a slow-paced walk, but you can try different speeds to see what works best for your attentiveness.

1. Select a place where you can walk 10 to 30 paces back and forth or in a circular pattern, or you can simply walk outside wherever you feel safe and comfortable.

2. Keep your hands at your side wherever they are comfortable.

3. Notice your surroundings.

4. Take a breath in and be aware of your feet on the ground and your body supported by the earth.

5. Start with a slow walk or a leisurely stroll, but be aware and in tune to your body.

6. With each step, notice how your foot moves, lifts, swings, and goes back to the ground.

7. Notice any other sensations that come up in your body and mind as you move.

8. Use your mindfulness of the present moment and your awareness of your body to stay connected to your movement.

9. Continue walking for 10 to 20 minutes, being aware of when your mind wanders off and gently bringing it back to your walking meditation.

As you become more comfortable with this type of walking awareness, you can use it in your everyday life. Wherever you go, mindful awareness is available.

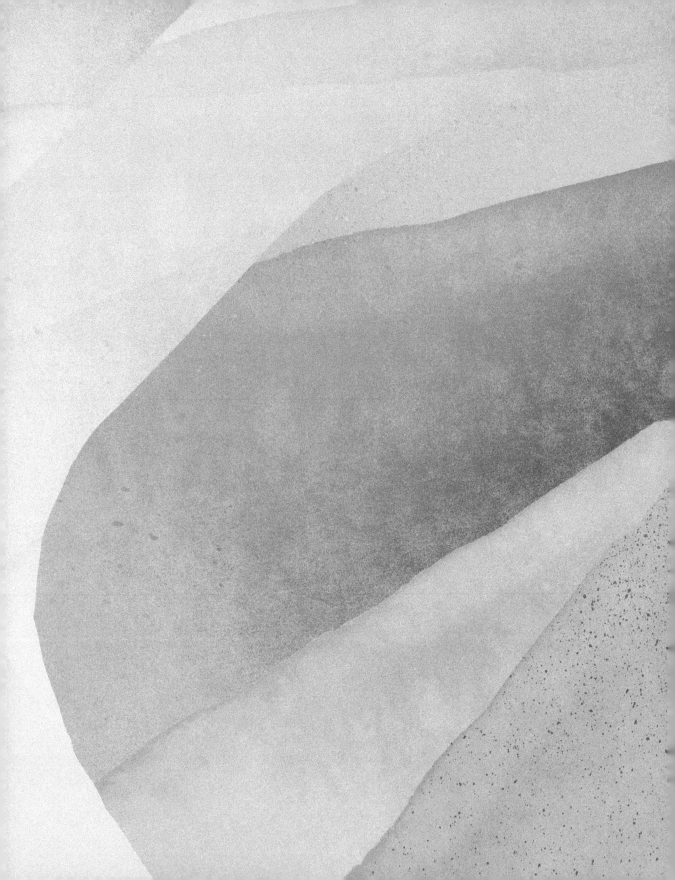

chapter seven

New Situation, New Strategies

Even if you've been pregnant before, it's important to remember that each pregnancy experience is different.

When you find yourself in a brand-new situation, you may experience new kinds of stress or have new reasons for feeling out of control. In these instances, finding a successful way to cope is essential. The skills you've used in the past may continue to work, and it's absolutely worthwhile to see if they do. However, sometimes they might not. That can be frustrating, but that doesn't mean *nothing* will work. Remember, you always have options.

In this chapter, we'll go over some different skills and tools to try, especially if you feel like you haven't quite found what works best for you in your pregnancy. The key in assessing if something is going to work for you is to try it out several times or for several days.

Remember that there's no rule about how many skills or tools you can accumulate. Gather all that you want, and use them to find what works best for you. Now, let's explore some strategies to help you take confident steps forward in your journey.

Butterfly Hug

This technique is used in eye movement desensitization and reprocessing (EMDR) therapy, which is a therapy used for healing the emotional distress that is a result of traumatic life situations (see page 26). The butterfly hug is a skill that is used for calming the mind and body and feeling grounded. When it's used to feel grounded and soothed, this skill employs slow bilateral stimulation (BLS), which is essentially alternately tapping each side of the body: left, right, left, right, and so on.

Containment

You don't always have time to deal with difficult emotions, thoughts, experiences, or sensations when they come up, especially during pregnancy when you don't know how your past experiences will interact with your new journey. And sometimes you don't want to deal with difficult feelings at all. It can be hard to know what to do with feelings of being overwhelmed if you're in the middle of doing something like working, driving, or shopping.

One tool to use is the visualized container, which helps build emotional regulation. When feelings of high stress arise, some people feel overwhelmed, as if their emotions are out of control or their only option is to sit with the great discomfort. You don't want to deny your feelings, but you also don't want to be taken over by them. The balance can be containing your feelings in a safe place, knowing that your experiences are important and will be addressed at a later time. Ideally, if you have a psychotherapist you are working with, you can utilize the container exercise in session or in a safe space with a trusted person.

Containment also helps increase the capacity to tolerate big feelings. Many times, with anxiety or trauma, people are worried that their experience will take over, so they feel compelled to avoid or ignore the feeling. That may work for a time, but inevitably, your feelings come back around. By using a container that you know you will encounter again, you can take the sting out of avoidance and learn how to address your feelings without being taken over by them.

Butterfly Hug

The butterfly hug helps regulate our physical and emotional stress and soothe overwhelm. It is important to do the bilateral movements in this exercise slowly and rhythmically in order to bring comfort to the mind and body.

1. Sit comfortably in a chair or on the floor. Keep your eyes closed or softly gaze at a point on the ground in front of you.

2. Take a couple of deep breaths.

3. Cross your arms over your chest, put your hands on your chest with your fingers below your collarbone, and interlock your thumbs, creating a butterfly shape on your chest with your hands.

4. With slow, deliberate taps that are not too hard and not too soft, begin tapping your chest one hand at a time, alternating at a pace no faster than every other second. One, pause, two, pause, three, pause, four, pause, five, pause, and so on.

5. Inhale and exhale, using a slower breath as you notice any sensations in your mind and body.

6. Continue this exercise for 30 seconds to 1 minute.

7. When you are done, take a moment to notice any sense of calm or relaxation that has come with the practice.

If you find that the butterfly hug is not comfortable or easy for you to do, you can cross your arms across your chest, with your hands touching your arms. Or you can rest your hands on top of your thighs and tap with these hand positions as well. You can even alternately tap your feet if that movement is what is most available to you.

Container Exercise

▼

Imagine a container, such as a box, storage bin, jar, chest, or basket of any color, texture, or shape you prefer. Its purpose will be to hold all of the thoughts, feelings, experiences, or sensations that you don't have the time or will to deal with in the moment. This container is meant to be a safe, secure, reliable place to hold whatever you need it to until you're ready to look at it again. You can imagine that it has a lid or door, a latch or key, or a handle to create a sense of safely storing something away.

Remember, the container is not for hiding these feelings or experiences or making them disappear. It is simply a place to safely and comfortably hold them until you want to address them.

1. Develop the container of your choosing in your mind.

2. Imagine placing anything in there that feels too overwhelming.

3. Take a breath.

4. If your container has a lid, lock, or latch, imagine securely closing it, knowing that you can open it when you want or need.

5. Imagine placing the container somewhere that feels safe to you where you can access it anytime you want.

Please be aware that you may have to continue to gently put things back in the container if and when they reoccur as an overwhelming sensation or thought. Accept that this will happen, and take comfort knowing that your job is to safely redirect those heavy feelings back to the container.

Journaling

There are an infinite number of benefits to journaling. After all, it is an expression of you and of your relationship with yourself. How often do you really sit down, allow yourself to think, write, type, reflect, review, and contemplate the processes of your own mind? With busy schedules and distractions, especially during a pregnancy, you likely don't get nearly enough time to really focus on and check in with yourself. Taking just 5 to 20 minutes a day to have time with yourself can greatly benefit your mental health by allowing you time to reflect, slow your mind and body, and release your thoughts and feelings. It also increases your capacity to think more deeply about your experiences.

Styles and modalities of journaling vary widely, from reflection and stream of consciousness to prompts about a specific topic, feeling, or situation. There is no right way or wrong way to journal. However, there is some research indicating that a positive focus (such as journaling about a time you succeeded or felt happy) rather than a negative focus (such as reflecting on a time you felt disappointed) has better mental health outcomes overall.

Benefits of Journaling

Journaling during pregnancy or when you're preparing for pregnancy has many potential benefits. You are on the brink of something entirely new, an adventure in growing a human, becoming a parent, and expanding your sense of self. It is all at once amazing, beautiful, scary, and common. Still, it is your unique experience. Here are just some of the benefits of journaling:

LETS YOU TAKE NOTE OF YOUR JOURNEY. There will be things that happen during pregnancy, birth, and having a newborn that you feel certain you'll remember no matter what, but the truth is that you'll forget some things. Journaling can serve as a reflective memento for you and a way to connect to your child in those early days.

MAKES YOU SLOW DOWN. Journaling also makes you slow down, which is especially important for managing anxiety. You simply cannot write as fast as your brain can think, so journaling coaches your anxiety process to slow down. If you write out your thoughts and feelings, you may notice that it gives you time to reflect and move through them more gently.

INCREASES YOUR SELF-AWARENESS. Writing can also increase your awareness of how you feel and what you think. You can look back on your entries and reflect on your experience.

LETS YOU TRACK THOUGHTS AND FEELINGS. Getting thoughts and feelings out of your head and on paper can help you know that your thoughts and feelings are somewhere, so you don't need to ruminate to keep track of them.

INCREASES YOUR ABILITY TO PROCESS DIFFICULTIES. You can process difficult situations, conversations, feelings, thoughts, and even physical issues through journaling. This is especially helpful if you can't talk to anyone else about it yet or need to sort things out for yourself before sharing.

HELPS RELEASE AND EASE SYMPTOMS OF ANXIETY. Journaling can help release and ease symptoms of anxiety. It's a method of validation to be able to acknowledge your own feelings and see them on paper, know that they are real, and know that it's okay.

Pointers for Journaling

When it comes to journaling, what is most important is that it works for you. The journal is a judgment-free zone where spelling and grammar don't really matter. Think of it as your space to freely express yourself.

YOUR JOURNAL CAN BE ANY STYLE YOU WANT IT TO BE. When you journal, you don't have to freewrite. You can use lists, drawings, words, quotes, or stories—whatever works for you.

YOUR JOURNAL CAN INCLUDE WHATEVER YOU WANT IT TO INCLUDE. Your journaling can focus on a specific topic, such as your path to pregnancy, the journey of your pregnancy, your changing mood, your dreams or goals, or what you are grateful for.

THERE IS NO RIGHT OR WRONG WAY TO BEGIN. Journaling can start with a specific daily or weekly prompt, such as "Today I am feeling . . ." or "I'd like to tell my baby . . ." or "This week I need to . . ." or "How I am really feeling . . ."

YOU CAN SIMPLY WRITE. Another approach is to just write. Don't think about the act of writing or focus on what might come next. Give yourself over to the process of freewriting. This is a powerful form of journaling because it allows your conscious mind to be an observer. You can learn a lot from yourself when you get out of your own way.

Additional Prompts for Pregnancy and Anxiety

If you need some assistance getting started, consider some of the following prompts to kickstart your journaling efforts.

- *What went well today?*
- *What is pregnancy like for me?*
- *How do I feel about the changes in my body?*
- *What are my fears and hopes for the pregnancy?*
- *What are my fears and hopes for the birth?*
- *How do I feel about becoming a parent?*
- *What kind of support do I want from my partner or family?*
- *What am I feeling worried about and what are ways I'd like to cope?*
- *What is going well in my pregnancy?*

When It's Not "Just" Anxiety

In my psychotherapy practice, the majority of my clients are pregnant or postpartum. Many clients are anxious and not totally sure why, or they know they are anxious but the skills they used to use are just not working. This is generally a flag for me to assess for trauma and post-traumatic stress disorder (PTSD). I've learned over the years that many people have experienced traumatizing situations but don't know that it was trauma. Some people grew up in an environment that was chaotic or unpredictable and figured out how to survive. But because their experience was happening daily, it seemed like just another day of the same. In other cases, people have experienced a situation that was traumatizing as a child or as an adult but haven't had support to understand it or work through its impacts.

Trauma is also not often assessed or recognized in general physician visits because doctors are not trained to catch it. They may not know what it can look like, but that's not their fault. Trauma and mental health haven't historically been addressed by medical healthcare providers.

In addition to going unrecognized, trauma is often minimized by others around us or by ourselves. Sometimes when people share stories of trauma,

My Journaling Prompts

Do you have any ideas of specific prompts or ways that you'd like to use journaling? Take time to consider what questions you would like to prompt yourself with and what you want to take into consideration when preparing to journal.

seeking understanding and support, they might receive a response that sounds like one of these:

- *It wasn't that bad.*
- *You're okay now.*
- *Well, at least X didn't happen.*
- *That was a long time ago.*
- *It was only X.*
- *Let it go already.*
- *Move on. You're fine.*

If you have received these types of responses from others or said these things to yourself, it doesn't necessarily mean that you've experienced a trauma. However, if you also have some of the trauma symptoms outlined in chapter 1, it would be worthwhile to consider assessment with a psychotherapist.

(You can look back to chapter 1 for symptoms of PTSD and anxiety to see if this distinction fits for you. These checklists are not meant to offer a diagnosis but rather to help you understand your experience and consider getting professional help if needed.)

When considering if it's trauma and/or anxiety, ask yourself these questions:

- Do you find yourself minimizing your experiences?
- Did you have difficulties in childhood or as an adult that continue to weigh heavy on your mind?
- Do you get very uncomfortable or feel numb when you hear or see something that reminds you of your own experiences?

Some specific considerations for pregnancy and unrecognized trauma can be related to previous pregnancy loss or a difficult birthing experience. Challenging childhood experiences can also arise in your thoughts or memories when you're pregnant or while interfacing with medical providers, if that has been your experience.

The good news is that trauma is treatable, and it doesn't have to feel heavy or difficult forever. There are many types of useful trauma psychotherapies that can help, which we'll now explore.

Reducing Expectations and Pressure

Hardly anyone knows what they're doing all of the time, and no one has absolute control over what is happening in their life. If you have anxiety or trauma, these statements might make you feel more anxious, but if you can accept them, you can experience incredible relief. Despite what anxiety may tell you, you don't have to know everything, and you don't have to be perfect. You need only remember that you learn as you go and do what you can, and that's enough.

I continue to feel surprised by the amount of pressure that pregnant people put on themselves. I blame some of it on society and social media holding pregnancy up as a pristine and glamourous experience. Yes, it can be, but I can assure you, it is also messy and very unglamorous.

In some ways, I wish the myths were true. Wouldn't it be lovely to be glowing and fulfilled, to know your purpose, to be so in love with your baby, to feel well physically, to be positive and happy and thrilled to be pregnant with a partner who dotes on you? Wouldn't it be nice to sit with your feet up while you get a massage and eat bonbons? Wouldn't you love to wear clothes that fit well, to have a picture-perfect nursery, and a baby that's born on the due date? That all sounds like a movie, which is part of the problem. Unrealistic standards like this set us up for feeling less than.

Pressures and expectations are sometimes related to perfectionist tendencies, not in regard to how you look or dress, although that can certainly be at play, but in how you internally expect perfection. What does it sound like in your head when you're judging yourself? Does it get really intense in there, like you need to put more pressure on yourself?

There is no research to date that says being hard on yourself and having high expectations helps you be a good parent. Our inner critic's high expectations aren't natural; rather, they're learned over time. While we are born with certain tendencies and genetic predispositions, we aren't born to berate ourselves. Somewhere along the line, whether it be from family, friends, or community, you learned to do this to yourself. I would just love for you to know that you don't have to. You can unlearn this.

Why don't we aim to become really comfortable with not being perfect?

Both/And

Your mind can perform shorthand thinking and distort your thoughts when you are stressed or worried. For instance, if you're set on having a vaginal birth, you might think, "Either I have a vaginal birth or I'm not doing what I'm supposed to for my child." But those two things aren't actually related. Two seemingly different things can be true at the same time. You can have a C-section and be doing great for your child. Pregnancy and parenthood can make you think in terms of either/or.

I often hear from clients who don't like being pregnant that there must be something wrong with them. In reality, you don't have to love pregnancy, and if you don't, that doesn't mean something is wrong with you. That is the either/or thinking talking. You can hate pregnancy and be excited to be a parent. You can love pregnancy and not be excited to be a parent. One way of feeling doesn't cancel out other ways of feeling. When you reconcile the opposites, a new truth emerges that is more representative of the whole experience.

If you find that your thoughts tend to generate negative possibilities, you can consider adding an "and" to balance them out. For instance, if you're in a situation where there is tension in your relationship and find yourself thinking, "My partner always forgets to ask me how I'm doing," consider if that is absolutely true. Then, reframe the thought to "My partner often forgets to ask how I'm doing and sometimes remembers to ask."

Another way you can hold two truths is to see someone's point of view but not agree with it. And if ever you feel stuck in your thinking, you can try to look at things from someone else's point of view to gain more perspective and clarity.

Let's Get Real, Then Dial It Down a Notch

▼

This exercise is meant to help you reflect on the ways in which you are hard on yourself, setting expectations that are too high or being overly self-critical. There are times when those tactics could be self-motivating, but pregnancy and the postpartum period are not that time. The perinatal period is a time of learning, growing, flexible thinking, accepting support, and being kind to yourself as you enter into parenthood. With the questions below, reflect on how you treat yourself.

- What are your expectations of yourself in pregnancy?
- What kind of pressure do you feel, either from yourself or from those around you?
- If you don't meet those expectations and pressures, what will happen?
- Is the worry about what will happen actually likely?
- What if you don't do things perfectly?
- Are there other possible neutral or positive alternatives to the outcome you're worried about?
- How could you care for yourself with more gentleness?
- If you were 5 percent less hard on yourself, what would that look like?

As you move through your pregnancy and on to new parenthood, reducing your expectations and pressure on yourself can ease some of that anxiety. This practice will also help immensely when the baby comes so that you can have more mental flexibility and ease as a parent.

Two (or More) Truths

▼

You can notice either/or thinking if you find yourself drawn to viewing situations and feelings in black-and-white terms, if you use words like *always* or *never*, or if your thoughts feel rigid or one-sided.

1. Do your best to notice these feelings and ideas, and write down your either/or thoughts.

2. Attempt to see what a possible compromise between them could be.

3. How can these two opposites both be true at the same time?

EITHER/OR		BOTH/AND
I don't like being pregnant, so I'm destined to be a bad parent.	→	I don't like being pregnant, and I will still be a good parent.

This tool will be useful in so many ways when you become a parent. Holding on to opposite truths enables you to be flexible in your thoughts, to compromise two or more truths, to see situations through a broad and encompassing lens, and to make way for acceptance. Parents deserve this kind of understanding as they learn and grow with the child.

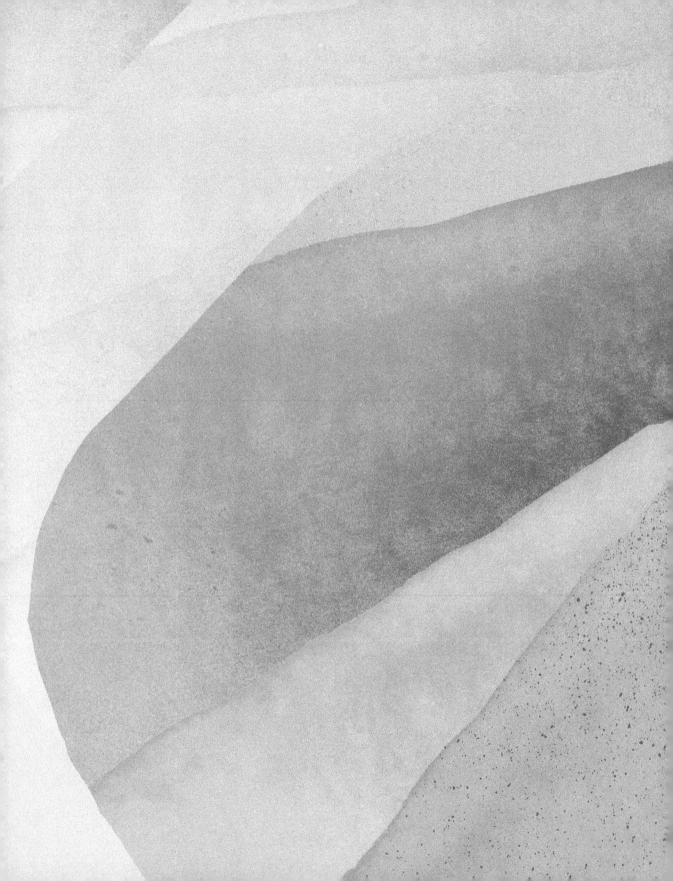

chapter eight

Anxiety and Postpartum

Many people worry during and after the birth of a baby. It's normal to be vigilant and concerned about your baby. Having a clinical diagnosis of an anxiety disorder is not the same thing as feeling worried about your newborn. Postpartum anxiety is more common than most people know, but it's not widely known about or discussed as openly as it could be. People may brush off clinical anxiety as new-parent worries. I can tell you from personal experience, postpartum anxiety can be rough, especially if you don't know what just hit you.

Anxiety, depression, panic, obsessive-compulsive disorder (OCD), post-traumatic stress disorder (PTSD), or any other mood condition can show up at any time in the first year after birth. It is a misconception that mood changes only happen in the early postpartum period. As we talk about postpartum conditions in this chapter, please keep in mind that they are very treatable. With the right kind of help, you can minimize the impact of postpartum mental health changes and reduce their intensity. It is incredibly helpful to have a psychother-apist set up before the postpartum period so that you have support in place for when you need it. Just knowing that support is available can minimize the intensity of your anxiety because you know that you're not alone.

When Anxiety Continues in Postpartum

Jasmine came in for psychotherapy at three months pregnant. She was experiencing worry, fear, and overwhelming feelings about her pregnancy, even though she was glad to be pregnant. Upon further assessment, her therapist discovered that she had experienced occasional anxiety symptoms throughout her life, but she was generally able to cope and live with them. In therapy, Jasmine learned several coping tools for anxiety, and by the middle of the pregnancy, she was feeling better and more able to cope. After the birth of her baby, she had a sharp increase in anxiety due to the birth experience and then moderate anxiety for another month or two. Jasmine wasn't able to feel very connected to her baby, even though she was doing most of the caregiving. It felt hard for her to believe that everything was going to be okay. During this time, Jasmine's coping skills weren't working as well as they had been. She sought out a reproductive psychiatrist for a medication evaluation. She started on a low dose of an SSRI antidepressant medication, and her symptoms resolved some several weeks later. After Jasmine felt better, she was able to reflect on how much the anxiety affected her capacity to feel connected to her baby. She felt that if she hadn't been to therapy during pregnancy, her postpartum might have been worse because she wouldn't have the skills and tools that she did. Having the support of someone who knew her already was also beneficial. Jasmine and her therapist had a postpartum plan set up to reduce some of her stressors. Having a solid care team in place helped minimize the intensity and duration of her symptoms and get her back to feeling like herself and growing as a parent with her baby.

If anxiety, OCD, PTSD, or panic started during pregnancy and was not treated, it is highly likely it will continue or worsen in the postpartum period. This is because all of the anticipation that is present while awaiting the arrival of the baby—the planning, wondering, worrying, hoping, fearing—comes to fruition when the baby is actually born.

If you seek treatment for anxiety during pregnancy, you may still experience anxiety symptoms in postpartum. There can be a sense of letdown or sadness that comes along with continued anxiety because it's another way that the experience of pregnancy, birth, or the postpartum period isn't what you may have wanted it to be. But if you have useful skills, tools, and support, you can be better able to cope and manage.

It is very hard to endure anxiety during pregnancy and then have it continue or worsen in the postpartum period. The hope for that anxiety to end when the baby comes is a very real hope. It can be disappointing or even devastating if you continue feeling the anxiety afterward.

When Anxiety Starts Postpartum

When I was a new parent, nighttime was the hardest for me. It felt like the third shift of the day. When my husband and I would get my daughter ready for bed, my anxiety would increase. She slept next to the bed in a co-sleeper and was in arm's reach at all times. I would fuss over how her swaddle was placed, worrying that it was too loose or too tight. I would lie awake in the dark looking at her to see if she was breathing and anticipating her waking up at any moment needing to nurse. I figured she would be up soon enough, so it would be easier to just stay awake than try to sleep. When she would finally wake up hours later, I would go to her immediately, nurse and change her, then hold her to get back to sleep. I'd fall asleep holding her only to wake up in a state of worry that she'd fallen over onto the bed. But she was always fine, perfectly content and asleep and safe. This nighttime routine went on for weeks, and I never told anyone that I was suffering with such intense anxiety.

The birth of a baby also means the birth of a new life for you as a parent. When navigating a new experience that naturally lends itself to nervousness, it can be difficult to know if you're having clinical anxiety or not, especially if the postpartum period is the first time you've experienced this kind of anxiety. Some people think that feeling anxious or overwhelmed is how all new parents feel because it's normal to have worries as a new parent, so they downplay their feelings.

If you felt good with regards to mood during your pregnancy, then developing a postpartum mood disturbance can be very upsetting. Sometimes the anxiety doesn't even register as actual anxiety but as an all-consuming feeling that makes you feel indescribably bad.

The range of conditions associated with anxiety that can emerge during pregnancy can also manifest in the postpartum period:

- Generalized anxiety
- Panic attacks or panic disorder
- OCD
- PTSD

You can look at the symptom checklists in chapter 1 to see if any of these categories might fit you. The checklists are not meant to offer diagnosis but rather to help you understand what is happening for you so that you can assess if it's time to get professional support.

Even though the postpartum period is a distinctly different time and context than pregnancy, the experiences have a lot of overlap.

Common Experiences of Continuation or Start of Anxiety Postpartum

When postpartum anxiety becomes more intense, it can begin to impact your day-to-day functioning. Your thoughts can feel like they are jumping all over the place, dominating your day with an unshakeable sense of worry. Often those worries are focused on the baby. You can feel constantly on edge and have difficulty feeling settled. Your vigilance can turn into hypervigilance, as you're constantly on the lookout to make sure nothing bad happens to the baby or to other people in your life. Your heart may race or pound in your chest. You may be unable to sleep even though you're exhausted. You might not have an appetite, or you might eat more often. You may feel generally overwhelmed and distressed. The anxiety may increase at nighttime and wake you up in the middle of the night, or you may feel anxious as soon as you wake up in the morning.

Birth plans and wishes play out as they play out and can contribute to stress. Depending on how the birth went, it can either contribute to a smooth transition or to continued anxiety or trauma. Anxiety related to the birth and postpartum period is influenced by many factors, including your health, the health of the baby, the birthing environment, the medical team, your support people, your home environment, and your partner or family.

SLEEP LOSS. Everyone's sensitivity to the effects of sleep loss is different; however, in postpartum, most everyone is affected. It is normal for babies to wake often throughout the night and for parents to wake right along with them. After several days of sleep loss, your brain and body lack the sleep and rest they need to function at full capacity. This can make you feel agitated, irritable, exhausted, less rational, or more anxious or depressed.

INABILITY TO SLEEP. Even if you're exhausted and need sleep, anxiety can keep you awake, your mind racing as you worry about the baby and all of the details of the day. If one parent is nursing or primarily responsible for feeding the baby at night, there is a particular dynamic that happens with high anxiety. That parent will sometimes not want to go to sleep because they anticipate having to wake up again soon to feed the baby. Sometimes the baby does wake up soon, but sometimes they don't. This reinforces the parent's pattern because sometimes babies do wake up sooner than expected, but when they don't, the parent is awake with their thoughts, maybe even researching their worries on their phone at 2 a.m.

HEARING EVERYTHING. Many anxious parents can hear a pin drop at night. Any little movement from the baby or little grunts or sounds can wake a parent from light sleep. When they're really anxious, some parents will watch the baby or the baby monitor to make sure the baby is okay all of the time. They may be worried that they won't wake up when the baby cries, even though they do wake up with the slightest of sounds. The difficulty here is that anxious parents sometimes don't wake easily because they are so exhausted from being hypervigilant. It's a difficult pattern for new parents because the worry comes from love, and the hypervigilance feels like care. It is care, but it comes from worrying something bad could happen.

CONSTANT WORRY. I see this in the eyes of the parents I meet who are gripped by anxiety. It's a feeling of not being able to settle or rest. They're always on the lookout, checking on the baby, worrying about anything that doesn't seem quite right. Are they eating enough? Sleeping enough? Warm enough? Cool enough? Peeing and pooping enough? What does this color of poop mean? Why are they making those sounds? Anxious parents are always wondering if their baby is okay.

FEELING OUT OF CONTROL. After a period of time, sometimes not that long, the anxiety can make you feel like you're on a hamster wheel and can't slow down. You may feel like something is wrong with you, but you're not losing it altogether. This is what anxiety and sleep deprivation can feel like. Getting sleep and getting help really can calm your nerves.

INTRUSIVE THOUGHTS. These are disruptive, disturbing, involuntary, and unwanted thoughts or images that pop into your head. For new parents, the thoughts are often about something bad happening to themselves, the baby, or someone they care about. These thoughts create their own anxiety and can feel scary. They can involve worry about harm or germs, may create doubt, or be violent or sexual in nature. Intrusive thoughts can happen with anxiety, PTSD, or OCD, but they also just occur sometimes. People do not want to act on those thoughts. They are actually usually repulsed by them. These thoughts don't mean anything about you or point to anything you are capable of. They generally result from your brain being on overdrive to protect your child, even though nothing bad is actually happening. Intrusive thoughts can often mean that your body is responding to a hormonal shift, that the anxiety is very high, or that you need to sleep or feel less stressed.

GRIEF. It is upsetting when the postpartum period and life with your baby do not turn out how you wanted, especially if you or your baby are experiencing any health conditions or complications or if you're having difficulty transitioning to parenthood. Anxiety conditions can particularly affect how you feel during that first bit of time with your child, even throughout the first year. If you're sad or feel like you lost out on a smooth transition to parenthood, you may be grieving that loss. It's okay to feel upset about that. It's hard to deal with.

There are other common experiences for postpartum anxiety conditions. Generally, if you're feeling something that you don't understand, you're not alone. It's not just you. Many other people are trying to cope with similar feelings. However, your experience is still unique to you and deserves support, understanding, and treatment as needed.

COLIC

Colic is a condition where the baby cries for several hours a day for several days a week for several weeks or more even when they are fed and healthy. This condition can contribute to and increase postpartum anxiety, depression, frustration, and overwhelm. Parents often try everything they can think of to ease the crying, such as going to the doctor, changing the baby's formula, or modifying what the nursing parent is eating. Sometimes parents are frustrated because care providers may only have a few strategies for helping the baby, or they may just tell the parents that the baby will eventually grow out of it. It's important to know that colic is not your fault. Some babies just have sensitive systems in the early months. Consult with your pediatrician, find a support group of other parents who are managing this, and ask your friends and family for help so you can get breaks for yourself.

Postpartum Anxiety versus Postpartum Depression

When you're feeling anxious after having a baby, it's hard to know when things will get easier, especially if you are a first-time parent. Experiencing anxiety after your baby arrives or anytime in the first year can be a major source of stress. The combination of stressors over time can intensify, especially if depression becomes a part of your experience.

Postpartum anxiety and postpartum depression often show up together, but one can precede the other. Long stretches of any kind of stressor can lead to depression or anxiety because it lingers longer than expected. Our stress response is meant to deal more effectively with short-term stress. However, in situations of prolonged stress or situations that don't have a clear ending point, like a pandemic for instance, it's hard for our brains and bodies to tolerate the stress and still feel balanced.

There are multiple factors that can contribute to postpartum mental health changes. The postpartum period brings major hormonal shifts in the first week after birth, and some people are more susceptible to the effects of those changes. Sleep deprivation, of course, is another culprit.

It's worthwhile to see if symptoms of depression are playing a part in your stress and overwhelm. Many people assume that postpartum depression means that you don't want to take care of the baby. While that can be a part of how it feels for some people, that's not how everybody feels. As a matter of fact, some people feel like the baby is the only thing keeping them going.

Symptoms of depression can range from mild to moderate to severe and can include the following:

- Low, sad, or down mood
- Not wanting to do things you used to do
- Feeling bad about yourself, feeling worthless or like you are letting people down
- Sleeping more or less than usual
- Eating more or less than usual
- Having little energy
- Difficulty concentrating
- Thoughts of death or suicide

BIRTH-RELATED TRAUMA

Sometimes birth doesn't unfold as expected. Even if the birth seemed relatively smooth to everyone else in the room, it may not have been the birth you wanted, or you may have had an emotional or physical experience that left you feeling traumatized. It can also be traumatizing if your baby needs to stay in the newborn intensive care unit after birth. In any case, if the birth of your child leaves you feeling traumatized or shaken up, know that those are valid feelings. No one else can tell you if you should feel traumatized or not as it is your experience. These kinds of birth experiences can leave people feeling worried and alone. Look in chapter 1 for symptoms of trauma to see if that could be what you're dealing with. You can absolutely feel better with the right help. Please consider psychotherapy with a therapist trained in perinatal mental health.

Screening for Postpartum Depression

▼

A common way to help screen for postpartum depression is the Edinburgh Postnatal Depression Scale (EPDS). This scale also incorporates some symptoms of anxiety. Completing this screening can help you figure out if you might be experiencing depression.

In the past 7 days:

1. I have been able to laugh and see the funny side of things.

- 0   As much as I always could
- 1   Not quite so much now
- 2   Definitely not so much now
- 3   Not at all

2. I have looked forward with enjoyment to things.

- 0   As much as I ever did
- 1   Rather less than I used to
- 2   Definitely less than I used to
- 3   Hardly at all

3. I have blamed myself unnecessarily when things went wrong.

- 0   No, never
- 1   Not very often
- 2   Yes, some of the time
- 3   Yes, most of the time

CONTINUED ▸

Screening for Postpartum Depression continued

4. I have been anxious or worried for no good reason.

    0   ⚪   No, not at all

    1   ⚪   Hardly ever

    2   ⚪   Yes, sometimes

    3   ⚪   Yes, very often

5. I have felt scared or panicky for no very good reason.

    0   ⚪   No, not at all

    1   ⚪   No, not much

    2   ⚪   Yes, sometimes

    3   ⚪   Yes, quite a lot

6. Things have been getting on top of me.

    0   ⚪   No, I have been coping as well as ever

    1   ⚪   No, most of the time I have coped quite well

    2   ⚪   Yes, sometimes I haven't been coping as well as usual

    3   ⚪   Yes, most of the time I haven't been able to cope

7. I have been so unhappy that I have had difficulty sleeping.

    0   ⚪   No, not at all

    1   ⚪   Not very often

    2   ⚪   Yes, sometimes

    3   ⚪   Yes, most of the time

8. I have felt sad or miserable.

    0   ⚪   No, not at all

    1   ⚪   Not very often

    2   ⚪   Yes, quite often

    3   ⚪   Yes, most of the time

9. I have been so unhappy that I have been crying.

    0   ⚪   No, never

    1   ⚪   Only occasionally

    2   ⚪   Yes, quite often

    3   ⚪   Yes, most of the time

10. The thought of harming myself has occurred to me.

    0   ⚪   Never

    1   ⚪   Hardly ever

    2   ⚪   Sometimes

    3   ⚪   Yes, quite a lot

Tally up the numbers. If your score is 10 or more, further assessment for depression is warranted. For men or people of color, a cutoff score of 8 or 9 respectively may be more accurate.

TOTAL SCORE _____

Coping Strategies

Learning how to cope with emotional overwhelm while you're learning how to be a parent can be a challenge. Parents these days have so much pressure to do more and be more for their children than ever before. With the pressures of social media and a million experts telling you what is best for each decision you have to make, it's no wonder that parents are overwhelmed. In this section, you can learn some mental and emotional tools for coping and managing the stress of the transition to parenthood. You might be surprised to hear that you can do less and still be a great parent. Being more present with your child and for yourself is good parenting, too.

Let Go of the List

People who are already dealing with anxiety before having a child can feel pressure after the baby is born to do all of the things they've always done plus all of the new things that come with parenthood. This is generally not sustainable. Care for a brand-new person isn't just related to tasks. A new parent also has an emotional process and needs to adjust to their new normal, figuring out what the baby needs, taking care of the baby, trying to take care of themselves, and so on.

The list of things to do can seem endless. Each new day brings new tasks or the need to redo the previous day's tasks: do the laundry, wash dishes, bottles, and pump parts, eat, shower, clean, and other daily tasks. This transition to having an increased number of tasks can be overwhelming. So much needs to be done, but much of the time with a baby is spent feeding them, changing them, getting them to sleep, or holding them for hours as needed. The list of tasks remains partially done or totally unattended to. Often, this leads to increased overwhelm, guilt, and anxiety that there is so much to still do. Everything feels like a priority. The challenge is to let go of doing everything on your list every day. Let's explore how you can do this:

1. Pick only one or two tasks a day as the goal.

2. If you get them done and have more energy and time to spare, then pick another task.

3. However, if you haven't eaten, drunk water, had a shower, or rested yet, then that one or two tasks you selected will be enough for the day.

4. The other things on the list can wait or be done by other people.

5. The list never ends, so you'll have a chance to do one or two more things tomorrow.

Lower Your Expectations

Try to take the pressure off of yourself to know everything about your baby, how to do everything they need and do it all well. New parenthood is largely trial and error with the best of intentions. Wanting to be a good parent is a great ideal, but it doesn't happen overnight, and perfection isn't possible. You're learning, your partner or family is learning, even the baby is learning. Nobody knows what they are doing or how to best support this particular baby, but you will figure it out with time. Lowering your expectations of yourself doesn't mean that you are going to be lazy or not take care of your baby. It means that you're going to be gentler with yourself and realize that it's okay to not do everything.

Anxiety in these early months is in some ways related to the pressure that parents put on themselves. If you ask most people how they got through the first three months postpartum, they'd probably say, "I don't know. I just did." Or they might admit, "I just had to figure it out along the way." Zero percent of people have ever said that they knew what to do all of the time with a newborn. I urge you to take a deep breath, lower your expectations of yourself, be gentle on yourself as you transition to parenthood, and keep trying to figure it out.

Good Enough

If you're worried that you aren't doing a good enough job as a new parent, that's a sign that you care a lot and are probably doing more than you think. It's also a possible sign of anxiety, depending on how worried you are and how much it's affecting you. I can't count the number of new parents I meet who are so worried that they aren't doing enough for their child that they absolutely can't see all that they are doing well. This anxiety doesn't allow for the normal learning process of parenting.

Anxiety makes us notice what we fear and magnifies it. So, guess what happens: Mistakes feel like failure. Not knowing what to do feels like being a bad parent. Needing a break feels like guilt. Not feeling like being a parent today feels like shame. But mistakes, not knowing what to do, needing a break, and not wanting to be a parent sometimes are totally normal. Our internalized ideals of

High Expectations

Time for some good old self-reflection again. Becoming aware of our patterns is key to learning how to cope differently. In this exercise, you can tune in and catch your negative self-beliefs and judgmental self-talk and then practice replacing them with a less emotionally charged assessment.

IF YOU CATCH YOURSELF SAYING THINGS LIKE . . .	Then, recognize that your thoughts and feelings are possibly a response to fatigue, overwhelm, pressure, or anxiety.	REPLACE THOSE THOUGHTS AND FEELINGS WITH . . .
I should know . . .		I'm doing my best right now.
I should be able to . . .		I'm learning.
Other people can. Why can't I? What's wrong with me?		We're learning.
This should be easier.		It's okay to not know what to do. I always figure it out eventually.
I don't know what I'm doing.		I am taking care of my baby.
I'm not doing enough.		
I'm not good enough.		It's okay if this feels hard. Other people struggle, too.
Your high expectations:		Thoughts to replace them with:

parenthood along with societal pressures tell us we are supposed to be grateful, in love, intuitive, all-knowing, and many other beautiful things.

The self-proclaimed failure of a parent and the lofty ideals of parenthood are two ends of a spectrum and, frankly, a setup for anxiety. There is an entire middle ground between the two, and most of us live there. Some bliss, some challenges, some mistakes, some wins—that can be a perfectly healthy balance.

If anxiety is affecting you in this way, chances are you might have difficulty seeing what you are doing well enough. Turning your attention to your strengths and wins for the day can help balance that out. If you can, go through a daily mental review of the things that were positive.

Getting Support

Getting support from friends and family does not mean that you are weak or incapable. It's important to dispel this myth upfront because if you carry this belief, getting support will make you feel guilty. Nobody needs that stress as they are figuring out parenthood. Becoming a parent does not have to be a one-person job, even if you are a solo parent. Create the village that you and your baby need in order to have as much ease, rest, care, and time for connection as possible. Support can take many forms. We will explore a few of them below.

Consider Your Circle

When thinking about what type of support you need from friends or family, you may think in terms of how close you feel to them, how much you trust them, or what kind of help they could offer. We all do this type of categorization with the people in our lives. For instance, you might be comfortable telling your best friend how you are really doing, but you might not want to tell your sibling that same information. But your sibling might be the person who will show up at your house when you're really in need of help. Or your coworker might be the person who will drop off food for you.

Negotiating Sleep

If there's one thing that you take away from this workbook, please let it be how important sleep is for your well-being. Sleep loss and deprivation is the number

Noticing the Good

In this exercise, you can practice awareness of what goes well in your day with your baby and with you personally. That might sound easy, but when you're fighting anxiety and stress, your brain is already attuned to the negative stuff. The negative is just easier to see when you're struggling. Making yourself notice the good is like building up your muscles, creating strength where you felt weak before. Take a couple of minutes or more every day to notice what is going well.

What went well for you today?

_____

_____

_____

_____

What went well for baby today?

_____

_____

_____

_____

What do you feel was easier today than it was a week ago?

_____

_____

_____

Make a list of all of the things you did today. (Hint: It's more than you think, so make an actual list.)

_____

_____

_____

Name three things that you can be grateful for today.

_____

_____

_____

What was good enough for today?

_____

_____

_____

one contributor that I see to worsened mental health in pregnancy and the postpartum period.

You're going to hear a lot of "sleep when the baby sleeps" from well-intentioned people. That sounds nice, but it's not often possible for a variety of reasons. By all means, if you can nap while your baby is napping, go for it. However, if you can't, you're not alone. Here's where negotiating sleep with a partner or family member comes in.

In the early postpartum stages, getting a stretch of more than three consecutive hours of sleep at a time is rare. If you're nursing the baby, then you're the primary source of food, which means you're up when the baby needs to nurse. If you have a partner or family member around, they can help with other things such as changing diapers and getting the baby back to sleep. If you're pumping or formula-feeding, then other people can step in for feeding.

If and when it's possible, negotiate hours for sleep. For instance, perhaps you can sleep from 8 p.m. to 2 a.m. while a partner or family member is the primary caregiver. They can sleep during that time, too, but they'll be the one to get up and take care of the baby when needed. Then, after 2 a.m., you're up and down with the baby the rest of the night while the other person sleeps. Ideally, you'd be able to get six hours of consecutive, uninterrupted sleep for several days in a row, then nap or rest when possible the rest of the day. Each person will need sleep for sure, but the birthing person is also healing and recovering, so at least in the first several weeks, you many need to renegotiate often. Please note that your baby's sleep pattern isn't settled or regular for several months. Growth spurts, teething, a cold, or any other change may disrupt their sleep and therefore yours. This is normal, but it is best if caregivers can be flexible with the sleep arrangements as issues arise.

Conversation Tips for Sleep Negotiation

- Talk with your partner or family members about which hours for sleeping work best for each of you.
- Consider who is going to be in charge of what for each set of hours (nursing, pumping, bottle-feeding, changing diapers, burping, etc.).
- How many days in a row can the birthing parent get consecutive hours of sleep? Come up with a weekly schedule if possible.
- Have a discussion about being flexible if these hours need to change or aren't working for either person.

Circle of Support

In the exercise below, think about the challenges you are having, the help you'd love to have, and who might be able to step in to support you. Then ask. It would be great if people could just know what you need and do it for you, but more often than not, we need to ask for that help. Sometimes people can help and sometimes they can't, so see if there's a backup person for the help you need.

Try to think if you need help just once or weekly or some other amount of time, and be as clear as possible when you ask. Reaching out for help can be hard to do, especially if you take pride in doing things yourself. Pregnancy and the postpartum period are different times. Asking for help isn't a sign that you're weak or can't do things. This is the time to call in the village. You'll have plenty of time to do everything yourself later.

What are your needs and who can help?

CHALLENGE	NEED	WHO MIGHT HELP	WHO CAN HELP
Groceries	Someone to bring food	Mom, cousin, friend	Cousin

- Do you need or want help from someone else? A grandparent, sibling, friend, postpartum doula, or night nanny?

Support Groups

Having a group of people who experience the same struggles you do can be incredibly validating. I've heard time and time again from support group members how relieved they are to know that they are not alone. Even if they can only partially relate to one or two people in the group, the group can become a safe place to be seen and heard. Some of my clients have stated that just one group meeting helped them know that they weren't the only one dealing with these issues. When they were home, feeling distraught and worried, they knew that group of other new parents would get it. There is a healing that comes from connection and the deep relief of validation.

When you're seeking group support, it's important to find one that fits you. Some mommy groups or new-parent groups might not talk about anxiety or depression. People may be connecting over the general stress of being a new parent but not discussing emotional or mental health changes. These groups can feel further isolating to people who are trying to cope with anxiety or depression.

Look for pregnancy or postpartum mental health groups specifically. You can even call and ask the facilitator what kind of group it is first. Searching the internet for postpartum support groups is a good place to start. You can look in the Resources section of this workbook for more suggestions on where else you can look for support.

When to Seek Therapy or Medication

There is no wrong time to seek out psychotherapy. You do not need to be suffering in order to get help. As a matter of fact, please don't wait until then if you don't have to. It's worthwhile to take the time to find a trained perinatal mental health professional. Many people struggle for too long, making bargains with themselves like, "If I just get some sleep, I'll be fine" or "It's not that bad. I don't need help." My professional and personal opinion is that you should get help or support before you need it, or at least if the thought pops into your head that you might need or want it.

Psychotherapy with a provider who is trained in perinatal mental health is beneficial if you're experiencing mild, moderate, or severe symptoms of anxiety, panic, OCD, or PTSD. A general rule of thumb is that mild symptoms are noticeable and cause some concern, but you can mostly cope through your day. Moderate symptoms will affect you more clearly. They are more disruptive to your day-to-day life and a cause for concern. Severe symptoms prevent or make it hard for you to get through the day and get in the way of regular daily activities like eating, sleeping, self-care, and functioning.

Seeking a medication evaluation or consultation from a reproductive psychiatrist, general psychiatrist, primary care provider, or nurse practitioner is fine to do at any level of severity. A medication evaluation would be suggested if you are experiencing moderate to severe symptoms that are not lessened by psychotherapy or are not resolving with sleep and support.

I'm a firm believer that knowing about potential perinatal mental health conditions beforehand is better than finding out about them by surprise. This workbook has a lot of information to look through, which can be overwhelming or produce more anxiety. I want to just call that out and let you know it's very normal to feel that way. There are so many great resources in the back of this book that can support you with prevention and healing. You can feel better with the right help and support.

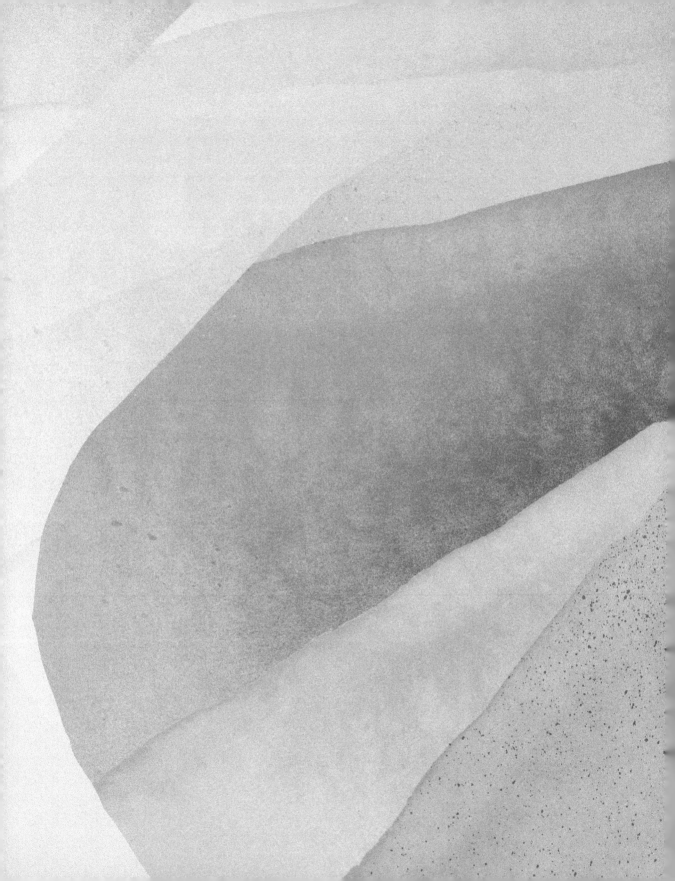

chapter nine

Doing It Together

Pregnancy, birth, and having a baby are life-changing experiences for not only the individual but also the partnership. Bringing a baby into a relationship changes the dynamics of the relationship and the types of issues partners communicate about. Although new parents now have a shared responsibility for the life of the baby, they may have different ideas about how to parent. About two-thirds of couples feel dissatisfied in their relationships after a baby is born. There are various reasons for this, but some include overwhelm from the work of parenthood, arguments over responsibilities, dealing with their own childhood issues coming up, fatigue, and over time, resentment.

I see this stress in couples who are having a difficult time, partly because there is much less time to communicate and connect. Planning ahead together for how you'll communicate and stay connected after the baby comes can help reduce some of this relationship strain. Still, these are ongoing conversations, so it's imperative that you regularly include time to communicate and connect.

Dear Partner,

Times may be different right now, possibly unsettling, scary, or overwhelming. As your partner continues along in their pregnancy, you're approaching a time of great change, steep learning curves, and adjustment to a new way of being in the world as a parent and a family. You and your partner may have different ways of approaching parenthood, preparing for the change, and parenting, and that's okay. Nobody knows what they are doing, but you will figure it all out along the way.

Before birth and during the recovery afterward, the birthing parent will experience a time of need that is essential to their well-being. More will be asked of you than you might have expected, but that's because you are essential to the health of the family as well. You will be going through your own adjustment to parenthood that may bring up feelings for you, and that's okay, too. I can assure you that this time will pass, and you will all get through this if you can find a way to stay connected and get support as needed. I hope to be able to help and support you here, too.

Sending patience and coffee,

Dr. Kat

Supporting Your Expectant Partner

In traditional families or those with culture-based gender roles, the mother births and nurtures, and the father provides and protects. When these roles are clearly defined, it's clear who is responsible for what (although that doesn't necessarily make it easier). However, in many Western, modern, or progressive households, both parental figures do everything, so shared responsibility has to be divided up differently. Many people who are attempting parenthood in this more egalitarian way may be doing so without the benefit of having learned how to from their own parents. How do you know what to do as a partner? How do you support someone who is pregnant and anxious? I'll offer some pointers and tips here that might be helpful to you both.

Communication between Partners

The first thing to know is that your partner might be anxious and possibly suffering, and you may not even be aware of it. There is a kind of anxiety that is very high functioning, so much so that it isn't apparent to anyone on the outside. The worry and stress are so internal that your partner might not even say anything about it. They're not necessarily trying to be secretive. They may just feel guilty or embarrassed or don't want you to think anything is wrong. They may want to be the pregnant person who feels great and may not really know how to cope with feeling anxious.

If your partner doesn't show how anxious they are, you don't have to ask them all of the time if they are okay. However, pregnancy is a great time to establish or strengthen your emotional communication. You're going to need it after the baby comes. Strengthening emotional communication is also good so that it's not a surprise to you if your partner isn't feeling well. If you're used to communicating about emotions and checking in with each other, that is great. It is important to continue to do so and not make assumptions about how the other person is doing.

If you are new to emotional communication, it can feel awkward at first. Just like any new endeavor, you may need to just do it and fumble through until you get your bearings. Once you begin communicating in an open and nonjudgmental way, over time, your partner will learn that they can talk with you about their worries and you'll still be there for them. The benefit is that this can go both ways. You can also share your worries and thoughts with your partner to get the support you might need.

If you've never dealt with anxiety or another mental health condition, you might not completely understand what your partner is going through. It might be hard to put yourself in their shoes, and honestly, you don't totally have to. But imagining what it might be like for them can help you have some compassion. If you can't imagine what it's like, you can just listen and believe their experience. You don't have to fix it, figure it out, or try to make them get over it, unless that is what they are asking for. Your role can simply be to listen and support.

Sometimes your partner's anxiety will be very noticeable. They may be on edge, talking about their worries, asking you for reassurance about any number of things, having a hard time resting, having panic attacks, crying frequently, or feeling a bit spacy or preoccupied with their thoughts. You may hear things that sound scary or strange from your partner—the thoughts they are having may be new and worrisome to them, too. They may tell you about scary thoughts or feelings they have, and if you can keep your cool and just tell them you're there for them, then you're doing pretty well. This is important because if you happen to respond in a way that makes your partner feel embarrassed, ashamed, or very misunderstood, they might not want to be as open with you. You might have a strong negative response to what they are saying or how they are feeling. It's important to take note of that. It's okay to express your concern and have your own feelings.

Be sure to talk about, and agree on, how to keep communication lines open and available. Sharing your thoughts and feelings in a safe and welcoming exchange really helps strengthen the relationship because you don't have to guess how the other person is doing. Sharing vulnerabilities and receiving each other's feelings with loving support strengthens your bond. It's important to show interest and concern. Your ability to be supportive can have a positive impact on their well-being and help them feel connected to you. After all, who wants to feel alone?

If your partner is experiencing anxiety, they cannot just snap out of it. If they could, they would have already. They don't want to be feeling the way they feel. It's very hard to be anxious and pregnant, and it's not something that you can just turn off. Just to be clear, I'm not saying that they can't get better. They can. However, they need the right kind of help, a supportive home environment, and a sense of being understood by you as much as possible.

Your partner's mental health and state of being can affect you as well. If the situation is stressful for a long period of time, it can wear you down. People affect each other, and you have feelings, too. It is possible for you to feel overwhelmed by their overwhelm. So, getting your own support through friends, counselors, or family can be an additional way to support your partner and your family.

Schedule Dates

▼

To help foster communication, you need actual time to communicate. With the busyness of life, it's common, if not easy, to move through the day or week without checking in with each other. It's important to build connection and communication time into your week. You and your partner can pick a time for a weekly date to enjoy intentional time together. This time can be open-ended, have a set minimum, have a specific agenda, or be honored however you see fit.

Here are some tips for setting time together:

- Mark the time on a shared digital or paper calendar.
- Make it the same day and time every week, or choose a different time each week based on both of your schedules.
- Decide whether you want to set an amount of time for the date or leave it open-ended. Try to spend at least 30 minutes together.
- Check in about how each of you is doing in general or related to the pregnancy.
- Think about what you like to do together or what you can use this time for.

Here are some ideas for what to do on your date: watch movies, play games, plan stuff for baby's arrival, make dinner, go on a walk or hike, talk about how you want to parent together, binge-watch a show, go on a picnic, take a drive, do a puzzle, take turns making breakfast in bed, or discuss worries or concerns.

How to Provide Support That Helps

Even when they're surrounded by family, friends, or loved ones, people can feel alone if no one is really trying to understand how they feel. Sometimes your presence is enough for support, but more often than not, what the pregnant person really wants is a partnership, a sense of togetherness and feeling understood. In fact, you both probably want that. It's helpful if you can support them in the way they prefer rather than in a way you assume works for them.

There are a couple of relationship challenges that I hear about quite a bit from the primary caregiver, who also sometimes ends up being the one who has to ask for help from the partner. To highlight this dynamic, I will use female pronouns for an example of what I hear in sessions.

Beginning in pregnancy and extending through the postpartum stage, the mother's partner assumes that she will ask for help when she needs it, so sometimes the partner simply doesn't offer help. Then the mom becomes upset because she always has to ask her partner for help, like setting up the crib or getting something ready for the arrival of baby. Her partner gets upset because they feel like the mom is nagging or controlling. Then there is an impasse. Mom doesn't feel comfortable or able to ask for help because of the pushback and begins to withdraw from the relationship and feel resentful. Her partner wants to feel wanted, needed, and helpful but doesn't want to be told what to do. They don't know what to do or how to help, so they begin to withdraw and become resentful as well.

One of the wishes I hear most often from pregnant and postpartum people is that they wish their partner would be able to see what needs to be done and just do it without having to be asked or told. You may not have this psychic ability; however, you can ask what your partner wants or needs support with.

These types of issues between couples are fairly common and can generally be avoided through a little bit of planning and asking. You don't have to figure it out on your own. Ask your partner what they want or need for support. See if it's something you can do. Allow yourself to fumble. You won't get it right every time, but the effort really counts.

Ways to Support Your Partner

ASK THEM WHAT THEY NEED. The way that you feel supported might be different from the way your partner feels supported. The way you give support may be different from how they give support. Taking the mystery out of how to support your partner can help reduce your stress, too. Ask them, "What can I do to help? Do you need anything?"

BE A LITTLE AHEAD OF THE GAME. Listen for the things that your partner says are bothering them or creating difficulty in their life. If there's something you can do to ease that for them, give it a try.

SHARE THE LOAD. The mental and emotional load of gearing up to be a parent starts early in pregnancy and often before. Your partner may be thinking of all of the things they and the baby will need during pregnancy and postpartum. You can be a part of that process as well because you are also gearing up to have a child. Figuring this stuff out together is part of early parenting.

SET REALISTIC TIMETABLES. If things need to get done around the house and you're the person to do them, figuring out when you can actually do those tasks and communicating that to your partner can be helpful. As your partner becomes more pregnant, they physically can't do as much as they could before. If they are waiting for you to do something so they can do the next thing after that, their anxiety might focus on the *when*. For example, if you can't set up the crib until the weekend, be as clear as possible about that timeline so your partner doesn't have to guess and can feel reassured knowing that it will get done.

HELP THEM GET HELP. If you or your partner are concerned about their mental health, help them find resources for support. You can conduct internet searches, call a provider, take them to appointments, and support them in finding a therapist, a psychiatrist, or both. Make an effort to educate yourself on the state of their mental health and what you can do to better understand and support them.

Signs Your Partner Is in Distress

Changes in your partner's behavior, especially warning signs that they could harm themselves or the baby, could very well signal that your partner is in distress and needs help.

It's very important to understand the difference between worrisome symptoms that need immediate attention versus symptoms that are distressing but not an emergency. If your partner is experiencing a mental health condition like anxiety, panic, post-traumatic stress disorder (PTSD), or obsessive-compulsive disorder (OCD), you may notice a change in how they behave, how they feel from day to day, or even how they interact with you or the baby. If you get a sense that something isn't quite right, be sure to listen. I hear too often that partners or family members blame a change in behavior on being tired or attribute any distress to the fact that the person just had a baby. It's easy to attribute some, if not all, behavioral changes to having a baby, but sometimes important signs are missed because they are easily dismissed.

Remember, your partner doesn't want to feel stressed, worried, or on edge, and they might not be aware of exactly what is going on. They might not even be outright telling you how they are feeling, but you may have a sense that something isn't quite right.

Let's look at some signs that your partner may need help.

Signs That Help May Be Needed

- Take note of the things that your partner is saying and doing. Sometimes they don't know what's wrong or how to fix things, but they may be unconsciously dropping hints that they are not okay. If you feel that they are a little different from how they used to be, don't be so quick to chalk it up to pregnancy moodiness, especially if it lasts for a couple of weeks or more.
- Listen for things like "I don't feel like myself," "I'm so tired/exhausted," "I'm not sleeping much," "My mind is racing," "I can't settle or sit down for long," "I'm worried about the baby," or "I don't want to do anything."
- Notice mood changes like irritability, frustration or overwhelm, sadness, worry, confusion, and emotional numbness.
- Notice behavioral changes like cleaning a lot, yelling, not letting anyone else care for the baby, repetitive behavior, constantly asking for reassurance, not being able to rest, not sleeping, sleeping excessively, not eating much, eating a lot more than usual, not being able to put thoughts together, checking on the baby a lot, or not checking on the baby at all.

Signs That Immediate Help Is Needed

- Not sleeping at all for a couple of days
- Saying or doing things that seem strange, odd, or out of character
- Seeming confused or disoriented
- Saying that they don't want to live or be here anymore or that they have an intent to harm themselves or the baby

- Saying that something is very wrong with the baby, but the baby is okay
- Not attending to the baby regularly, but they don't realize it
- Saying that they hear or see things that are not there

What to Do

- Talk with your partner. Tell them about your concern and that you want to help them feel better.
- Stay with them or have someone stay with them 24/7 until they can get help.
- Call their medical or mental health providers. Let them know what's happening and ask for guidance.
- If there is an imminent risk, take them to the emergency room.
- OCD intrusive thoughts are not an emergency.
- When in doubt, reach out to providers or to Postpartum Support International, which has a helpline and can support you in finding local resources.

How to Take Care of Yourself

Remember that you matter in this process, too. Yes, the birthing parent is going through the bulk of the physical, hormonal, and mental changes while pregnant. But you're going through your own changes, too. Your hopes, expectations, worries, fears, insecurities, and dreams for your child all may be part of what you're reflecting on.

It's a bit of a balancing act to tend to your partner's pregnancy anxiety and your own well-being. The more invested you are, the more you care, and so the more it may affect you. Taking care of your well-being is actually helpful to your partner. Relationships succeed when both people are doing well or when one person can hold steady for the other. Your partner can return the support when you need it also.

It's okay to feel well when your partner isn't. You don't need to suffer together in order to go through the experience together. What's most important is to validate your partner and be there for them as best you can. If they are wishing that they felt well, too, you can continue to support them as they heal and recover from their own journey through anxiety.

Reflect on Your Partner's Well-Being

Taking a moment to really notice how your partner is doing can be challenging while you're also preparing for or taking care of a baby. However, you have an important role in noticing any changes or indicators that your partner is having difficulty. The following questions are related to important mood-related symptoms. Think through the questions and take note of any changes you see so that you can help your partner get support from you, other family members, or a care provider.

- Have you noticed a change in their behavior, mood, or ability to function?
- What is their mood like? Is that normal for them?
- Have they been sleeping and eating?
- Have you had concerned thoughts about their well-being?
- How do they feel about the pregnancy or about the baby? Are you concerned about that?
- Does it seem like they are checked out or can they be present?

Self-Care Reflection

Use the following prompts to reflect on what you need for your self-care and stress management. You may not have had to think in these ways before having a child. Being intentional about noticing what helps you feel less stressed may feel new, especially when you're thinking about who you feel supported by. Check in with yourself with these prompts, and remember to come back to them every once in a while.

- What activities do you enjoy?
- Who do you reach out to when you're going through a rough patch?
- What helps you feel better when you're tired or burned-out?
- What helps you feel calm?
- What helps you feel energized?
- Do you need alone time or time to connect with others to feel replenished?
- How much sleep do you need and are you getting it?
- Do you eat regularly or as much as your body needs?
- Where does the bulk of your stress come from—work, home, or family?
- What boundaries with friends, family, or partners could help you feel better?
- Do you have any plans, activities, or dates to look forward to?
- How often do you need to be with friends or family for connection time?

Your Transition into Parenthood

When was the last time someone asked you how you are doing in your journey to becoming a parent? When was the last time you checked in with yourself about how you are doing? As the pregnancy progresses, take some time, either weekly or monthly, to really dive into what this experience is like for you. Get in touch with your worries and hopes for your life as a parent. Usually, the non-birthing parent is not showered in attention and care in the same way that the birthing person is. Some partners feel left alone or that they don't matter as much now that there's a baby on the way.

Your Own Anxiety

Partners can also experience mood changes like anxiety, depression, OCD, PTSD, and panic related to pregnancy and birth. Adoptive parents or any person who is partnered with a birthing person can experience these changes. The statistics and research need more bearing out for male and female partners; however, studies show that expecting dads have a 10 percent likelihood of developing paternal postpartum depression, and that number can go up to 50 percent if the birthing partner is depressed.

If you have a previously diagnosed anxiety disorder, your likelihood of developing anxiety again during times of stress is higher. Don't be afraid; just be aware. For partners, anxiety might not show up in the same way as it did in the past. It may be more focused on the pregnancy or the worry that something feels out of your control. When both partners are suffering, it can be very hard on both the individual and the relationship. When you both need help but can't quite be there for each other, it can feel isolating. If this happens, it's even more important for both of you to find support from a reliable and caring network of friends, family, and psychotherapy.

Any skills or tools that you've learned in the past could be helpful to put to use now, but since the anxiety about pregnancy and becoming a parent is potentially different from what you've experienced in the past, this situation might require a different skill set.

Check-In on Anxiety

▼

If your pregnant partner is experiencing anxiety, it may be harder to check in with yourself about your own anxiety. Partners will often set aside their own feelings or not even notice them in order to make space for the pregnant person's struggle. If you have a history of anxiety or are noticing that you're not quite feeling like yourself, it's worthwhile to pay attention to your own mental health so that you can get the support you need.

- What are the typical signs for you that anxiety is present?
- Do you have physical sensations?
- Do you have thought changes?
- Do you experience daily changes in sleep, eating, or socializing habits?
- What are the tools you've used in the past to help you cope?
- Do you feel like you can recall those skills now and use them?

Postpartum Anxiety in Partners

Anxiety, depression, panic, and OCD can flare up or develop during pregnancy if you've had any of these conditions in the past. These conditions can also present after the birth of a baby, especially if the birth was anxiety producing or traumatizing for you. As stated before, you have a risk of postpartum mood changes even if your partner is doing okay. If they are struggling, you're more likely to struggle as well.

The arrival of a new baby is a big transition. You just don't know how you'll feel or how it will affect you until that day comes. And like your partner, you may experience symptoms right away or anytime in the first year. As a matter of fact, some research shows that male partners' symptoms present more frequently in the three-to-six-month range.

You have feelings and are entitled to have a reaction to life changes as much as the next person. Mental health is highly stigmatized, and pregnancy and postpartum have additional pressures that are seen as women's issues. This societal myth around masculinity is actually hurting men and male-identified people. Perinatal mental health issues affect the family and partners, too.

If you're concerned your symptoms and experience are pointing to anxiety, OCD, or trauma, check out the checklist of symptoms in chapter 1. You can also complete the Edinburgh Postnatal Depression Scale in chapter 8.

If You've Come This Far . . .

Partner, you get points for reading and considering all of this information. Your involvement and care are critical to your and your family's health and wellness.

It is my sincere hope that this workbook offered some insight, skills, tools, aha moments, or a life raft for you on your journey through pregnancy and on to parenthood. Here are a few key takeaways:

- Sleep is magic.
- You're doing better than you think.

- Help is available from someone who really understands.
- You are not alone.

I hope at some point in the future you can reflect on your journey and see how capable you really are.

Partner's Wellness
Is Important, Too

▼

The following questions are aimed to help you hone in on feelings, thoughts, or symptoms that you may be having. If you notice any heightened response or feelings in relation to a question, it may be worthwhile to take a closer look at how you're doing.

- How are you sleeping?
- Are you eating regularly?
- Do you find yourself worrying a lot or having intense thoughts?
- Are you having scary, unwanted, and/or intrusive thoughts about you or someone else doing something that harms your baby?
- Do you check on the baby often because you're worried? Or do you feel like you're avoiding being around the baby?
- Do you find yourself drinking more or using other types of substances?
- Are you on your phone or playing video games more often than you used to?
- Do you feel irritable, frustrated, overwhelmed, or angry?
- Are you feeling resentful toward your partner?
- Does it feel like you don't know what to do and detaching feels more comfortable?
- Do you feel the need to work or leave the house more than usual?

There are some really great resources out there for partners to help cope with overwhelm and stress. You don't have to suffer through this alone. I know it's hard to reach out for help as the partner, but if you connect with a provider who's trained in perinatal mental health, they can provide you with the right help.

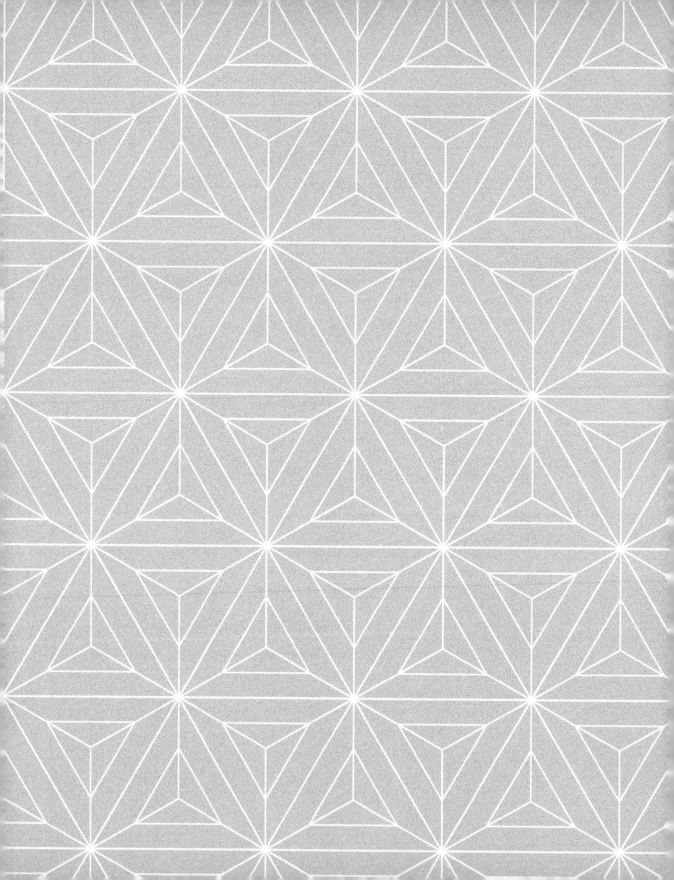

RESOURCES

Books

Beyond the Blues: Understanding and Treating Prenatal and Postpartum Depression & Anxiety by Shoshana S. Bennett and Pec Indman

Pregnancy Brain: A Mind-Body Approach to Stress Management during a High-Risk Pregnancy by Parijat Deshpande

The Recovery Mama Guide to Your Eating Disorder Recovery in Pregnancy and Postpartum by Linda Shanti McCabe

What No One Tells You: A Guide to Your Emotions from Pregnancy to Motherhood by Alexandra Sacks and Catherine Birndorf

Good Moms Have Scary Thoughts: A Healing Guide to the Secret Fears of New Mothers by Karen Kleiman and Molly McIntyre

And Baby Makes Three: The Six-Step Plan for Preserving Marital Intimacy and Rekindling Romance after Baby Arrives by John M. Gottman and Julie Schwartz Gottman

Happy with Baby: Essential Relationship Advice When Partners Become Parents by Catherine O'Brien

Tokens of Affection: Reclaiming Your Marriage after Postpartum Depression by Karen Kleiman and Amy Wenzel

The Postpartum Husband: Practical Solutions for Living with Postpartum Depression by Karen Kleiman

Training in Perinatal Mental Health

Any provider who works with pregnant, birthing, or postpartum people can train to become certified in perinatal mental health.

Postpartum Support International (Postpartum.net): Online and in-person training

The Postpartum Stress Center (PostpartumStress.com): Advanced training and small group training with expert Karen Kleiman

Seleni Institute (Seleni.org): Online and in-person training

Maternal Mental Health Now (MaternalMentalHealthNow.org): Self-guided online training

Education and Advocacy

Helpline: 1-800-944-4773 (#1 en Español or #2 English)

Text in English: 800-944-4773

Text en Español: 971-203-7773

Postpartum Support International (Postpartum.net): The leading national and international organization supporting parents, families, and professionals through group and peer support, education, and training and advocacy for perinatal mental health.

Perinatal Mental Health Provider Directory (PSIDirectory.com): A national directory of mental health providers who are trained in perinatal mental health

Perinatal Mental Health Alliance for People of Color (PMHAPOC.org): An organization focused on bridging the gaps between people of color and perinatal mental healthcare

2020 Mom (2020Mom.org): An organization that advocates for maternal physical and mental health

Maternal Mental Health Leadership Alliance (MMHLA.org): An organization that seeks to bring awareness to maternal mental health issues

PATTCh (PATTCh.org): An organization dedicated to the prevention and treatment of traumatic childbirth

Black Women Birthing Justice (BlackWomenBirthingJustice.com): An organization (and a book) that promotes birth and social justice for Black women

Black Mamas Matter Alliance (BlackMamasMatter.org): A maternal mortality and health movement

Every Mother Counts (EveryMotherCounts.org): An organization that works to make pregnancy and birth safe for all people

March of Dimes (MarchofDimes.org): An organization that works to improve the health of mothers and babies

Queer Birth Project (QueerBirthProject.org): A group of LGBTQ-identified birth and postpartum professionals

National Perinatal Association (NationalPerinatal.org): An organization that promotes evidence-based practices in perinatal care

Support for Pregnancy and Newborn Loss

Jessica Zucker (DrJessicaZucker.com): Author and creator of the #ihadamiscarriage awareness campaign

Return to Zero: H.O.P.E. (RTZHope.org): Support for families who've experienced pregnancy loss

Sisters in Loss (SistersInLoss.com): Support for Black families who've experienced pregnancy loss

Angels Born Still (DrIvyLove.com): Support and therapy for perinatal loss

Shoshana Center (ShoshanaCenter.com): Support, training, and therapy for perinatal loss

Star Legacy Foundation (StarLegacyFoundation.org): Information and resources for pregnancy loss

Medication during Pregnancy and Breastfeeding

Postpartum Support International (Postpartum.net): Free reproductive psychiatry consult line for medical providers needing consultation about medication for patients in the perinatal period

Massachusetts General Hospital Center for Women's Mental Health (WomensMentalHealth.org): Information and research on women's mental health

MotherToBaby (MotherToBaby.org): Information on medication during pregnancy and breastfeeding

Infant Risk Center (InfantRisk.com): Information and articles on medication risks during pregnancy and breastfeeding

Resources for Dads and Information on Paternal Postpartum Mood

Postpartum Support International (Postpartum.net/get-help/help-for-dads): A variety of resources for postpartum fathers

The Center for Men's Excellence (MenExcel.com): A group of therapists who focus on improving men's mental health

Will Courtenay (WillCourtenay.com): A therapist who specializes in men's mental health

Social Media

@postpartumsupportinternational
@momandmind
@postpartumstress
@momgenesfightppd
@healthy.highriskpregnancy
@pregnancyafterlosssupport

@sarahoreckmd
@shadesofblueproject
@drsayida
@corazoncounseling
@indigenousmotherhood

Podcasts

Mom & Mind
The Fourth Trimester
Motherhood Sessions

The Motherly Podcast
Delivering Miracles
Sisters in Loss

REFERENCES

Abramowitz, Jonathan. S., Samantha Meltzer-Brody, Jane Leserman, Susan Killenberg, Katherine Rinaldi, Brittain L. Mahaffey, and Cort Pedersen. "Obsessional Thoughts and Compulsive Behaviors in a Sample of Women with Postpartum Mood Symptoms." *Archives of Women's Mental Health* 13 (2010): 523–30. DOI.org/10.1007/s00737-010-0172-4.

Abramowitz, Jonathan S., Stefanie A. Schwartz, Katherine M. Moore, and Kristi R. Luenzmann. "Obsessive-Compulsive Symptoms in Pregnancy and the Puerperium: A Review of the Literature." *Journal of Anxiety Disorders* 17, no. 4 (2003): 461-78. DOI.org/10.1016/S0887-6185(02)00206-2.

American Psychiatric Association. *Diagnostic and Statistical Manual of Mental Disorders: DSM-5*. 5th ed. Washington, DC: American Psychiatric Association, 2013.

Aron, Elaine. *The Highly Sensitive Person: How to Thrive When the World Overwhelms You*. New York: Harmony Books, 2016.

Ayers, Susan, and Elizabeth Ford. "Posttraumatic Stress during Pregnancy and the Postpartum Period." In *The Oxford Handbook of Perinatal Psychology*, edited by Amy Wenzel, 182-200. Oxford: Oxford University Press, 2016.

Beck, Cheryl T. "Panic Attacks during Pregnancy and the Postpartum Period." In *The Oxford Handbook of Perinatal Psychology*, edited by Amy Wenzel, 150-66. Oxford: Oxford University Press, 2016.

Beck, Cheryl T. "The Slippery Slope of Birth Trauma." In *Motherhood in the Face of Trauma. Integrating Psychiatry and Primary Care*, edited by Maria Muzik and Katherine Lisa Rosenblum, 55-67. Cham, Switzerland: Springer, 2018. DOI.org/10.1007/978-3-319-65724-0_4.

Bennett, Shoshana, and Pec Indman. *Beyond the Blues: Understanding and Treating Prenatal and Postpartum Depression and Anxiety*. N.p.: Untreed Reads Publishing, 2019.

Bronfenbrenner, Urie. *The Ecology of Human Development*. Cambridge: Harvard University Press, 1979.

Deshpande, Parijat. *Pregnancy Brain: A Mind-Body Approach to Stress Management during a High-Risk Pregnancy.* Self-published, 2018.

Dhillon, Anjulie, Elizabeth Sparkes, and Rui Duarte. "Mindfulness-Based Interventions during Pregnancy: A Systematic Review and Meta-analysis." *Mindfulness* 8 (2017): 1421-37. DOI.org/10.1007/s12671-017-0726-x.

Fairbrother, Nichole, and Jonathan S. Abramowitz. "Obsessions and Compulsions during Pregnancy and the Postpartum Period." In *The Oxford Handbook of Perinatal Psychology,* edited by Amy Wenzel, 167-81. Oxford: Oxford University Press, 2016.

Fairbrother, Nichole, Patricia Janssen, Martin M. Antony, Emma Tucker, and Allan H. Young. "Perinatal Anxiety Disorder Prevalence and Incidence." *Journal of Affective Disorders* 200 (2016): 148-55. DOI.org/10.1016/j.jad.2015.12.082.

Fawcett, Emily J., Nichole Fairbrother, Megan L. Cox, Ian R. White, and Jonathan M. Fawcett. "The Prevalence of Anxiety Disorders during Pregnancy and the Postpartum Period: A Multivariate Bayesian Meta-analysis." *Journal of Clinical Psychiatry* 80, no. 4 (2019): 18r12527. DOI.org/10.4088/JCP.18r12527.

Gottman, John. M., and Julie Schwartz Gottman. *And Baby Makes Three: The Six-Step Plan for Preserving Marital Intimacy and Rekindling Romance after Baby Arrives.* New York: Three Rivers Press, 2007.

Goyal, Madhav, Sonal Singh, Erica M. S. Sibinga, Neda F. Gould, Anastasia Rowland-Seymour, Ritu Sharma, Zackary Berger, et al. "Meditation Programs for Psychological Stress and Well-Being: A Systematic Review and Meta-analysis." *JAMA Internal Medicine* 174, no. 3 (2014): 357–68. DOI.org/10.1001/jamainternmed.2013.13018.

Grigoriadis, Sophie, Lisa Graves, Miki Peer, Lana Mamisashvili, George Tomlinson, Simone N. Vigod, Cindy-Lee Dennis, et al. "Maternal Anxiety during Pregnancy and the Association with Adverse Perinatal Outcomes: Systematic Review and Meta-analysis." *Journal of Clinical Psychiatry* 79, no. 5 (2018): 17r12011. DOI.org/10.4088/JCP.17r12011.

Hoge, Elizabeth A., Eric Bui, Luana Marques, Christina A. Metcalf, Laura K. Morris, Donald J. Robinaugh, John J. Worthington, et al. "Randomized Controlled Trial of Mindfulness Meditation for Generalized Anxiety Disorder: Effects on Anxiety and Stress Reactivity." *Journal of Clinical Psychiatry* 74, no. 8 (2013): 786-92. DOI.org/10.4088/JCP.12m08083.

Kleiman, Karen. *Good Moms Have Scary Thoughts: A Healing Guide to the Secret Fears of New Mothers.* N.p.: Familius, 2019.

Kleiman, Karen. *The Postpartum Husband: Practical Solutions for Living with Postpartum Depression.* N.p.: Xlibris, 2000.

Kleiman, Karen, and Amy Wenzel. *Tokens of Affection: Reclaiming Your Marriage After Postpartum Depression.* New York: Routledge, 2014.

Kwon, Rachel, Kelly Kasper, Sue London, and David M. Haas. "A Systematic Review: The Effects of Yoga on Pregnancy." *European Journal of Obstetrics & Gynecology and Reproductive Biology* 250 (2020): 171-177. DOI.org/10.1016/j.ejogrb.2020.03.044.

Linehan, Marsha M. *Cognitive-Behavioral Treatment of Borderline Personality Disorder.* New York: Guilford Press, 1993.

McCabe, Linda Shanti. *The Recovery Mama Guide to Your Eating Disorder Recovery in Pregnancy and Postpartum.* London: Jessica Kingsley Publishers, 2019.

Mennitto, Serena, Blaine Ditto, and Deborah Da Costa. "The Relationship of Trait Mindfulness to Physical and Psychological Health during Pregnancy." *Journal of Psychosomatic Obstetrics & Gynecology,* May 13, 2020. DOI.org/10.1080/0167482X.2020.1761320.

Misri, S., J. Abizadeh, and S. Nirwan. "Depression during Pregnancy and the Postpartum Period." In *The Oxford Handbook of Perinatal Psychology,* edited by Amy Wenzel, 111-31. Oxford: Oxford University Press, 2016.

Muzik, Maria, Susan E. Hamilton, Katherine Lisa Rosenblum, Ellen Waxler, and Zahra Hadi. "Mindfulness Yoga during Pregnancy for Psychiatrically At-Risk Women: Preliminary Results from a Pilot Feasibility Study." *Complementary Therapies in Clinical Practice* 18, no. 4 (2012): 235-40. DOI.org/10.1016/j.ctcp.2012.06.006.

Nhat Hanh, Thich. *No Mud, No Lotus: The Art of Transforming Suffering.* Berkeley: Parallax Press, 2014.

O'Brien, Catherine. *Happy with Baby: Essential Relationship Advice When Partners Become Parents.* N.p.: Higher Shelf Publishing, 2020.

Paulson, James F., and Sharnail D. Bazemore. "Prenatal and Postpartum Depression in Fathers and Its Association with Maternal Depression: A Meta-analysis." *JAMA* 303, no. 19 (2010): 1961–69. DOI.org/10.1001 /jama.2010.605.

Puryear, Lucy J. *Understanding Your Moods When You're Expecting.* New York: Houghton Mifflin, 2007.

Sacks, Alexandra, and Catherine Birndorf. *What No One Tells You: A Guide to Your Emotions from Pregnancy to Motherhood.* New York: Simon & Schuster, 2019.

Schwartz, Jeffrey M. *Brain Lock: Free Yourself from Obsessive-Compulsive Behavior.* 20th anniversary ed. New York: Harper Perennial, 2016.

Shapiro, Francine. *Eye Movement Desensitization and Reprocessing (EMDR) Therapy: Basic Principles, Protocols, and Procedures.* 3rd ed. New York: Guilford Press, 2018.

Wenzel, Amy, ed. *The Oxford Handbook of Perinatal Psychology.* Oxford: Oxford University Press, 2016.

Wenzel, Amy, and Karen Kleiman. *Cognitive Behavioral Therapy for Perinatal Distress.* New York: Routledge, 2015.

INDEX

A

Acceptance and commitment therapy (ACT), 26
Acupuncture, 39
Advice, dealing with unwelcome, 29
All or nothing thinking, 59
Anxiety
    day-to-day sources of, 68, 70
    feelings of vs. clinical diagnosis, 6–7
    infertility, 4
    physical signs of, 17
    pregnancy, 2–3
    pregnancy loss, 4
    symptoms, 8
Aron, Elaine, 53

B

Birth, worries about, 34, 36
Birth plans, 36
Birth-related trauma, 148
Birthing centers, 39
Body changes, worries about, 33–34, 35
Body scan, 121–123
Both/and thinking, 137, 139
Boundary-setting, 29
Breathing techniques
    breath counting, 102, 104
    diaphragmatic breathing, 100–101
    square breathing, 102, 103
Bronfenbrenner's ecological systems theory, 66–67
Butterfly hug, 128, 129

C

Caffeine, 111
Catastrophic thinking, 61

Chiropractors, 39
Cognitive behavioral therapy (CBT), 26
Cognitive distortions, 58–64
Colic, 147
Communication
    about feelings, 18–23
    between partners, 165–167
Compulsions, 15, 48–49, 86–87. *See also* Obsessive-compulsive disorder (OCD)
Containment, 128, 130
Coping skills
    for anxiety spirals, 38
    butterfly hug, 128, 129
    containment, 128, 130
    identifying, 46
    journaling, 131–133, 134
    postpartum anxiety, 152–155

D

Dates, scheduling, 167
Depression, 39, 49, 89
Disqualifying the positive, 61
Domestic violence, 52
Doulas, 37

E

Edinburgh Postnatal Depression Scale (EPDS), 149–151
Emotional reasoning, 59
Emotions. *See* Feelings and emotions
Environmental stress, 65–67
Exercise, 110
Exposure and response prevention (ERP), 49, 88
Eye movement desensitization and reprocessing (EMDR), 26

F

Family
 postpartum support from, 155, 159
 sharing feelings with, 21
Feelings and emotions
 about the path to pregnancy, 32–33
 anxiety, 6–7
 awareness of, 71–75
 expressions of anxiety, 13–15
 mindfulness with difficult, 119–120
 sharing with family, 21
 sharing with friends, 22
 sharing with partners, 18–20
Fight, flight, or freeze response, 13
Friends
 postpartum support from, 155, 159
 sharing feelings with, 22

G

Grief, 146
Grounding technique, 54
Guided imagery, 102, 105–106

H

Hanh, Thich Nhat, 120
Healthcare providers, 37, 39
Highly sensitive persons (HSPs), 53
Hospitals, 39

I

Infertility, anxiety in, 4
Internet research, 36–37, 76–77
Interpersonal psychotherapy (IPT), 26
Irritability, 14

J

Journaling, 131–133, 134
Jumping to conclusions, 62

L

Lactation consultants, 37

M

Maternal mental health
 psychotherapists, 37
Medications, 26, 40–42, 161
Meditation
 about, 114–115
 barriers to, 115–117
 benefits of, 113
 body scan, 121–123
 guided imagery, 102, 105–106
 during pregnancy, 115
 sitting, 118–119
 walking, 124–125
Mental filtering, 63
Midwives, 37
Mind-body connection, 17
Mindfulness
 about, 114
 barriers to, 115–117
 benefits of, 113
 coloring, 118
 with difficult emotions, 119–120
 with difficult thoughts, 120–121
 during pregnancy, 115
Miscarriage. See Pregnancy loss

N

National Coalition Against Domestic
 Violence, 52
National Domestic Violence
 Hotline, 52
Naturopathic doctors, 39
No Mud, No Lotus (Hanh), 120
Noticing the good, 156–157
Numbness, 15
Nurse midwives, 37

O

Ob-gyns, 37
Obsessive-compulsive disorder (OCD)
  intrusive thoughts, 82–88
  and pregnancy, 47–50
  and psychosis, 88
  symptoms, 9–10
Overgeneralizing, 60
Overwhelm, 15

P

Pain, birth, 36
Panic and panic attacks
  defined, 7
  as an expression of anxiety, 14
  intrusive thoughts, 88
  and pregnancy, 43–46
  symptoms, 8–9
Parenthood
  beliefs about, 68, 69
  expectations about, 153–155
  transition into, 174
Partners
  anxiety in, 174–175
  communication between, 165–167
  intimate partner violence, 52
  postpartum anxiety in, 176
  self-care for, 171, 173
  sharing feelings with, 18–20
  signs of distress in pregnant,
    169–171, 172
  support for pregnant, 165, 168–169
  wellness considerations, 177
Pelvic floor physical therapists, 39
Perinatal mental health specialists,
    24–28, 37
Personalization, 63
Postpartum anxiety
  about, 141–144
  coping strategies, 152–155
  experiences of, 144–147
  in partners, 176

vs. postpartum depression, 147–151
  professional help for, 160–161
  support for, 155, 158–160
Post-traumatic stress disorder (PTSD)
  intrusive thoughts, 88
  and pregnancy, 50–54
  symptoms, 10–11
Pregnancy
  anxiety in, 2–3
  beliefs about, 68
  expectations about, 136, 138
  feelings about the path to, 32–33
  medication and, 40–42
  and obsessive-compulsive
    disorder, 47–50
  and panic attacks, 43–46
  and post-traumatic stress
    disorder, 50–54
Pregnancy loss
  anxiety in, 4
  mindfulness and meditation for, 117
Pregnancy support groups, 37
Prenatal massage, 39
Professional support, seeking,
    24–28, 160–161
Progressive muscle relaxation
    (PMR), 107–109
Psychosis, 89

R

Rage, 89
Relationships. See Family; Friends; Partners
Relaxation techniques
  about, 99
  breathing, 100–102, 103–104
  exercise, 110
  fresh air, 110–111
  guided imagery, 102, 105–106
  music, 111
  prenatal yoga, 110
  progressive muscle relaxation, 107–109
  rest, 111

Reproductive psychiatrists, 37
Rest, 111
Restlessness, 14

S

Schwartz method, for OCD
    treatment, 49–50
Self-compassion, 16
Self-doubt, 14
Sex (assigned) of baby, worries about, 34
"Should" thinking, 62
Sleep, 43, 145, 155, 158
Social media, 76–77
Stressors, 65–67, 71–77
Support groups, 160

T

Therapists, 24–28
Thoughts
    acceptance of, 91–92
    avoidance of, 93
    awareness of, 71–75
    both/and, 137, 139
    catastrophic/worst-case scenario, 14
    distraction from, 91

    identifying and labeling negative, 58–64
    identifying and labeling scary, 90
    intrusive, 7, 14–15, 48, 80–87, 146
    and mental health conditions, 88–89
    mindfulness with difficult, 120–121
    obsessional, 15, 83–85
Thyroid function, 41
Tokophobia, 36
Trauma, 51–52, 133, 135, 148.
    See also Post-traumatic stress
    disorder (PTSD)

V

Visualization, 120–121

W

Walking, 110, 124–125
What if? thinking, 60, 95, 96
Wise mind technique, 5
Worry, 14, 146
Worry time, 93–94

Y

Yoga, prenatal, 110

ACKNOWLEDGMENTS

Thank you to my awesome husband—without you stepping up at home and encouraging me, this book wouldn't be possible.

To my daughter and son, whenever I think I can't love you more, then I do. Thank you for being excited for me and patient when I couldn't watch movies with you.

Thank you to my mom and dad for the support, encouragement, and belief in me, which seem endless. Thank you to my brother and family, who always have my back, cheer me on, and make me laugh.

To my dear friend and colleague Dr. Long, my best friend Delanie, my therapist Mary, and my mentor Keri, thank you for encouraging me and helping me break past the mental and emotional barriers to writing.

To my clients who show up, dig deep, and do the work of healing, your strength is inspirational. Your healing is a joy.

To all of the hopeful and new moms, dads, and parents out there, I had you in mind while writing. I truly hope this book supports you in your journey to parenthood.

ABOUT THE AUTHOR

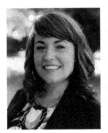 **Katayune Kaeni**, Psy.D., PMH-C, also known as Dr. Kat, is a psychologist who is certified in perinatal mental health and specializes in the assessment and treatment of perinatal mood and anxiety disorders. She works with clients in person and online through her clinical practice Well Mind Perinatal. Dr. Kat serves on the board of Postpartum Support International as executive committee member-at-large and chairs the certification, education, and training committee. She is the creator and host of *Mom & Mind*, the only podcast of its kind to focus solely on perinatal mental health through shared personal stories and expert interviews. You can find out more about her at DrKaeni.com, MomandMind.com, @momandmind on Instagram, and @momandmindpodcast on Facebook.

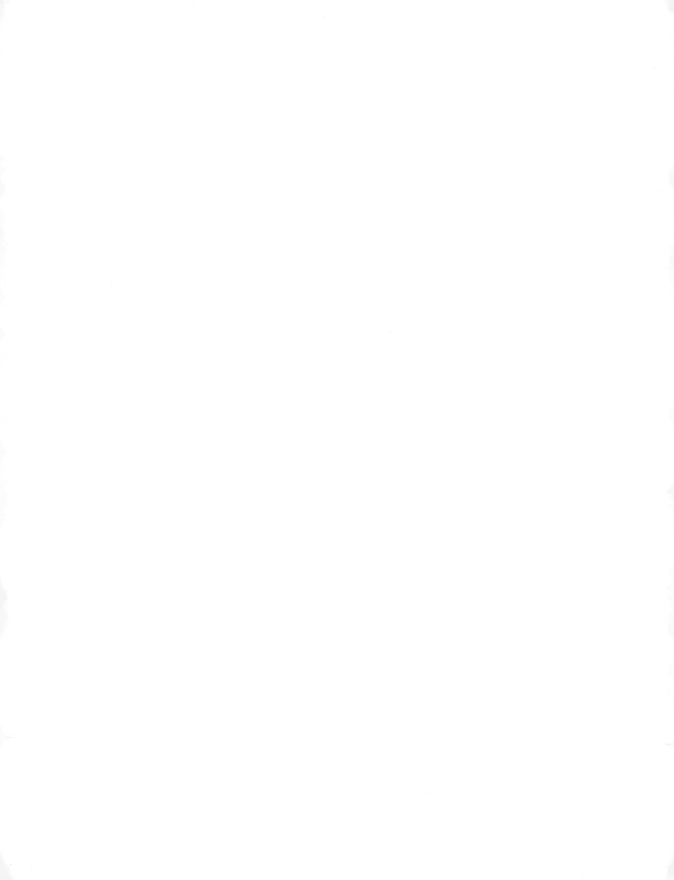

Printed in the USA
CPSIA information can be obtained
at www.ICGtesting.com
JSHW042334230923
48732JS00002B/2

9 781648 768378